A Holistic Approach to
VIRUSES

David Brownstein, M.D.

For further copies of **A Holistic Approach to Viruses**
Call: **1-888-647-5616** or send a check or money order in the amount of:
$25.00 ($20.00 plus $5.00 shipping and handling) or for Michigan
residents $26.20 ($20.00 plus $5.00 shipping and handling, plus $1.20
sales tax) to:

Medical Alternatives Press
4054 Oak Bank Ct.
Orchard Lake, Michigan 48323

ISBN: 978-0-9840869-7-9
Medical Alternatives Press
4054 Oak Bank Ct.
Orchard Lake, Michigan 48323
(888) 647-5616

Acknowledgements

I gratefully acknowledge the help I have received from my friends and colleagues in putting this book together. This book could not have been published without help from the editors—my wife Allison, Angela Biggs, and Clifford Scholz.

I would also like to thank my patients: Your search for safe and effective natural treatments is the driving force behind holistic medicine. You have accompanied me down this path, and I appreciate each and every one of you. Your acceptance of my treatment for COVID-19 was humbling.

And, to my staff: Thank you so very much for taking this trip with me. Without your help and support, none of this would be possible. I appreciate all your hard work and your dedication. And, especially during the misery and stress of COVID-19, I cannot thank you enough for your help.

A Word of Caution to the Reader

The information presented in this book is based on the training and professional experience of the author. The treatments recommended in this book should not be undertaken without first consulting a physician. Proper laboratory and clinical monitoring are essential to achieving the goals of finding safe and natural treatments. This book was written for informational and educational purposes only. It is not intended to be used as medical advice.

ABOUT THE AUTHOR

Dr. David Brownstein, M.D., is a board-certified family physician who utilizes the best of conventional and alternative therapies. He is the Medical Director for the Center for Holistic Medicine in West Bloomfield, Michigan. He is a graduate of the University of Michigan and Wayne State University School of Medicine. Dr. Brownstein is a member of the American Academy of Family Physicians and serves on the board for the International College of Integrative Medicine. He is the father of two beautiful physicians, Hailey and Jessica, and is a retired soccer coach.

Dr. Brownstein has lectured internationally about his success using natural therapies. He has also authored sixteen books: *Iodine: Why You Need It, Why You Can't Live Without It, 5th Edition; Vitamin B12 for Health; Drugs That Don't Work and Natural Therapies That Do, 2nd Edition; The Miracle of Natural Hormones, 3rd Edition; Overcoming Thyroid Disorders, 3rd Edition; Overcoming Arthritis; Salt Your Way to Health, 2nd Edition; The Guide To Healthy Eating, 2nd Edition; The Guide to a Gluten-Free Diet, 2nd Edition; The Guide to a Dairy-Free Diet; The Soy Deception; The Skinny on Fats; The Statin Disaster;* and *Ozone: The Miracle Therapy; and Heal Your Leaky Gut.*

Dr. Brownstein's office is located at:
Center for Holistic Medicine
6089 W. Maple Rd.
Suite. 200
West Bloomfield, MI 48322
248.851.1600
www.drbrownstein.com
www.centerforholisticmedicine.com

Contents

DEDICATION

To the women of my life: Allison, Drs.(!) Hailey and Jessica, with all my love.

To physicians not satisfied with the dogma, who are willing to search for a new paradigm that promotes health.

To my staff: Thanks so much for all of your help and encouragement. I appreciate all of your hard work.

And, to my patients. Thank you for being interested in what I am interested in. For trusting my care during COVID-19—I am (finally) at a loss for words!

Preface

The entire world is in crisis mode over a virus that harms very few people yet is sensationalized in the media as if it were the truly dangerous "Spanish" influenza that took many millions of lives worldwide. There is a runaway train headed for coronavirus vaccination, and likely mandatory vaccination.

Your immune system has needs. For example, take a neglected nutrient – iodine. Most people know it as required for thyroid function. But did you know it is required for proper white blood cell function in generating a crucial enzyme called myeloperoxidase? Vitamin C (ascorbic acid or ascorbate) is a well-known requirement for a host of biological processes. And, when you are ill, your body needs higher amounts to rise to the occasion, sort of like your engine needing heavier oil when running in hot weather.

One nutrient not discussed at length in this book is zinc. A deficiency of this mineral can lead to immune dysfunction, and if imposed upon lab animals, a subtle immune deficiency can be passed on to offspring for generations, even if the offspring are replete in zinc.

Another way your body is designed to fight an illness is your body's propensity to quell inflammation, and even suppress reactive coagulation. (Heightened coagulation can be a negative response to infection, clearly seen in the current coronavirus epidemic.)

Not all factors that regulate your immune response can be covered in a book, and not all factors that affect your immune system are even known. But what is known is that how you take care of your body DOES impact your immune response. You don't have to be "deficient" in a nutrient to have a problem. A better question is, "What is the optimum for me?" or: "What steps can I take to enhance my overall health instead of treating disease?" The conventional medicine of today waits for you to fall ill, then treats you as if you have a genetic deficiency of a synthetic petrochemical pharmaceutical. Does this make any sense?

The first order of business for me and my patients is to clean up what is likely a toxic diet (Standard American Diet or SAD). An emphasis on plant-based diet, organic, grown nearby if possible, ripe, not cooked to oblivion, is a first step, as it is rich in minerals and key nutrients. The next is to detoxify their bodies by any number of methods, from saunas and sweats, to exercise, to bowel cleansing, to heavy metal removal, etc. Toxins impair your body's adaptive response to stress and poison your enzymes, inhibiting repair, healing and defense.

The integrative/functional physicians will use targeted nutrients to optimize their patients' healing and defensive prowess. Simply being in the "reference range" in a lab test might be totally insufficient, as, for example, "normal" vitamin D levels can vary from say 30-100 ng/ml. Do you want yours at 30? I don't want mine that low, and despite lots of sun in sunny California, even my summer vitamin D level is in the lower end of this range. So, I do take supplemental vitamin D, as well as iodine–because this nutrient is not easy to get.

This book emphasizes four key nutrients, vitamins A, C, D and iodine, to optimize your response to viral challenges. This simple, but forward-thinking and actually peer-reviewed, published approach, makes far better sense than sitting back and letting a nutritionally compromised system try to mount an effective defense, or thinking that synthetic pharmaceuticals can replace what Nature requires for the best immune response.

Then there is oxidation therapy, which includes ozone and hydrogen peroxide. Did you know that a few pennies worth of hydrogen peroxide in 1918 nearly halved the death rate from viral pneumonia? You will read about that here. In 1944, another oxidation therapy (ultraviolet blood irradiation) was reported to cure 100% of 15 cases of viral pneumonia. Today, over 75 years later, conventional medicine has no specific treatment for viral pneumonia. However, ozone therapy, in widespread safe use for well over 100 years, has been conclusively proven to improve immune function. It is widely considered to be an ideal antiviral treatment. Studies on ozone indicating that it can greatly assist even hospitalized coronavirus patients have been recently published. Ozone remains the only published therapy which appears to be a cure for Ebola, the most lethal virus the world has ever seen.

Vaccines traditionally have been made by inactivating the virus for administration to activate an immune response to viral antigens. In the current crisis, there is a "warp speed" move for vaccination, and several paths are leading to a first–injecting you with viral genetic material, either RNA or DNA, so that your body will use the template to generate viral proteins and mount an immune response. However, this foreign genetic material could get incorporated into our own genome with disastrous consequences in the long run. In the experience of the integrative physician, it is far easier and more effective to treat a disease itself than attempt to treat the damage of vaccine injury. The pundits are rushing towards vaccination with all its unknowns– including medical problems that may not be known for years. Consider that asbestos exposure takes many years to manifest its injury.

Please remember a mantra of the integrative healer. "Provide your body with what it needs to do what the Creator designed it to do." The lessons in this book are an excellent first step in the current virus "crisis".

Robert Jay Rowen, MD
2200 County Center Dr. Ste C
Santa Rosa, CA 95403
www.drRowendrSu.com

Foreword

What makes a healthy immune system? Nutrients. Oxygen. Rest. How do we know this?

Basic biology. While complex, the innate and adaptive immune systems signal and work together to provide rapid, emergency responses to new pathogens and old, using the tools provided by natural selection over eons of time. Our innate immune system acts as a sentinel system, ready to respond at a moment's notice to intruders. The healthy cell death associated with innate immune killer cells that detect infections sets off a number of important signals that the adaptive immune system picks up, gets to work, and begins to produce cells that tags other cells infected with the virus, entire pathogens (in the case of bacteria), or foreign proteins.

When the FDA approves a drug, or affords a treatment Emergency Use Authorization (EUA), it relies on the ability of those making the proposal to show that it has efficacy (in the case of FDA approval) or may have efficacy (in the case of emergency use authorization). The treatment's ability to "work" can be measured in many ways; i.e., it may alleviate or reverse symptoms, reduce the symptoms of a disease, send a recurring condition into remission, or reverse the course of the disease and help a person become healthy again. A drug's use for a given condition might suggest utility in other uses, so-called "re-purposing," and these new applications are allowed in medicine under the concept of off-label use. A treatment should directly address the mechanism of disease; a therapy helps the body get better.

Sometimes the body can be its own worst enemy and overreact to a pathogen. The signals given off by an immune reaction can sometimes lead to a storm of intercellular signals known as cytokines. This is referred to as a cytokine storm. Sometimes the body's reaction can go haywire and lead to inflammation, or runaway processes that are pathological. This can lead to tissue destruction if the immune system attacks one's own tissues, or provoke other symptoms such as weakening of blood vessels, leakiness of blood vessels or in the case of COVID-19, an error in the signals to coagulate or to prevent coagulation of blood.

At the time of this writing, the exact mechanisms by which the virus SARS-CoV-2, the virus that causes the illness COVID-19, are still being discovered. We know that people who do poorly and progress to serious or critical illness and death are those with chronic inflammation or those with an autoimmune-predisposed immune system where Th2 cells outnumber Th1 cells: "Th-2 skewed". Some of these subjects appear to have proteins from other pathogens and remnants of cells from other pathogens in their blood, consistent with inflammatory bowel disease and leaky gut syndrome.

I have known Dr. David Brownstein for about four years, remotely, and now much better both personally and professionally, as we have worked together to make sense of COVID19. David called me early in the outbreak, and we discussed how some people were dismissing the gravity of the situation. "It's scary," he told me, leaving no doubt that we were on the same page about the potential harm from the virus. At the time, medicine only had clues from China on potentially effective treatments, which included a consensus statement on the utility of hydroxychloroquine. The Chinese reported that hydroxychloroquine had a high likelihood of being effective–along with various types of traditional Chinese herbal remedies. There was increasing information coming to light about the potential utility of selenium and zinc in helping to block viral entry. I asked David how he was handling the virus clinically,– and he relayed his practice's standard treatment for respiratory illnesses. He did not sound confident. "I hope it works," he said. "Me too," I said.

A month and a half later, David called and told me that the FTC had sent him a letter telling him that his online publication of video testimonies of patients who had received the therapy was a violation. "Why?" I said.

"They say 'because there is no study' supporting the therapy," was David's reply.

He had come to the right guy. I am an expert in basic clinical and translational research, and I am committed to objective science at all costs.

"How many patients have you helped, David?".

"Over one hundred" was his reply.

"So let's give them a study!" I suggested.

I invited him to consider publishing a case series study– the first phase of clinical research–to the journal *Science, Public Health Policy & the Law*, where I am Editor-in-Chief. We have a few papers published so far, and I knew that if the study had merit, it should be published.

"Okay!" Dr. Brownstein replied, enthusiastically.

"I'll be going with the reviewer recommendations" I reminded him.

"I know. Let me get to work on it" he said. And the rest is history. His study, "A Novel Approach to Treating COVID-19 Using Nutritional and Oxidative Therapies," survived three rounds of peer review by three practicing physicians and one Citizen Reviewer–a person representing the public, whose interests are underrepresented in the process of science and its publication.

The paper is still one of only a handful of studies available on COVID-19 treatment.

The consecutive case series, which describes the health outcomes of 107 patients under his care for COVID-19, provides a great deal of detail on the known mechanisms of action of the parts of the therapy Dr. Brownstein and his colleagues provide. This book fleshes out the rest.

The US Food and Drug Administration should take note: There is no reason not to issue an Emergency Use Authorization for this protocol for COVID-19, and there are 107 reasons why the EUA should be proffered. Obviously, as a case series, the study falls short of being a randomized clinical trial, but it certainly provides a solid basis for the next translation phase, with more science when it is compared to other protocols being used and being given consideration. I would like to see a multi-center trial conducted by individuals who are not stakeholders in any particular treatment, and who have no stake in the vaccine game. Such a study should be conducted ASAP to provide knowledge for the sake of knowing.

We know that healthy immune systems help people recover from infections. It is about as simple as that. Now let Dr. Brownstein tell you all of the why's and how's.

James Lyons-Weiler, PhD
Allison Park, PA

Chapter 1

Why A Holistic Approach

Why A Holistic Approach

I attended medical school from 1985–1989. In the course of my studies I was taught how to diagnose disease and pathology and how to prescribe drugs to treat various conditions. This is exactly what I did when I began my medical practice in 1992. Six months later, I started to realize that I was not helping my patients improve their health. The medications I had been taught to use did not, in the vast majority of cases, treat the underlying cause of the illness affecting the patient. In fact, the medications were causing other problems, requiring more drugs to control the problems caused by the first ones. This led to an uneasy feeling. I knew I had to find a better way to approach my patients.

Nowhere in my medical training was I taught about what health is or how to maintain it. Instead, I had become an expert on diagnosing pathology and prescribing drugs.

The drugs I was prescribing presented another problem. Nearly all pharmaceutical drugs work by one of two mechanisms: either they poison enzymes, or they block receptors in the human body. After nearly 30 years of practicing medicine, I can assure you that the long-term use of pharmaceutical drugs that block receptors or poison enzymes does not promote health. Instead, they cause a gradual decline in overall health and immune system function.

So, what is health? Health is much more than the absence of disease. A healthy person has adequate energy levels to perform whatever tasks they need to perform each day. This healthy individual's brain is strong and sharp from morning until bedtime. He or she will report feeling generally good most of the time. And, a healthy person, when confronted with a pathogenic illness, will have an immune system that responds appropriately by neutralizing and removing the pathogen from the body. After the illness is resolved, a healthy person will resume feeling well and go back to their previous energy and activity levels.

When I realized that the therapies I was taught in my medical training were not helping my patients achieve their optimal health, I began to search for a new paradigm.

My father, Ellis, was my first patient I treated holistically. Ellis had suffered his first heart attack at age 40 and a second one at age 42. Over the next two decades, he had two coronary artery bypass surgeries and angioplasties. At the time I completed my residency, my father was taking 12 different medications to treat heart disease, hypertension, high cholesterol and diabetes. Ellis did not feel well, as he suffered from continual angina for 20 years. To manage chest pain he was taking nitroglycerin pills like candy.

My first exposure to anything alternative in relation to medicine was through a chiropractor, Dr. Robert Radtke. He gave me a book, *Healing With Nutrition*, written by Jonathan Wright, M.D. In that book, I read how an allopathic physician was using nutritional and holistic modalities to treat his patients. I was intrigued.

Based on what I read in that book, I asked my father to come into the office. I drew his blood to be tested for testosterone and thyroid hormone levels. Ellis' testosterone levels were below detectable limits and thyroid hormone levels were in the lower reference range. Based on those tests, I placed Ellis on two natural supplements: natural testosterone and desiccated thyroid hormone.

Within seven days the 20-year angina symptoms resolved and never returned. My father began to look and feel better. Thirty days later his cholesterol level, which had been stuck in the 300's mg/dl range, fell below 200 mg/dl, without changing his bad habits. Seeing these dramatic improvements in my father's condition, I knew that this was the type of medicine I wanted to practice in order to help patients achieve their optimal health. I left the conventional practice where I worked and began practicing holistic medicine. Since treating my father, every patient I see gets a hormonal and nutritional evaluation. More information about my father's case can be found in my book, *The Miracle of Natural Hormones, 3rd Edition.*

When I began to check my patients for their hormone and nutrient levels, I saw that most were lacking basic nutrients and had hormonal imbalances. Correcting these imbalances by using natural therapies began to improve my patients' health. As I learned more and more about how to ensure that the body has the correct balance of nutrients, I saw my patients continue to improve their health status. Now, when I prescribe any therapy, I contemplate how it will affect not only the condition that brought the patient to my office, but the patient's health status overall. This is the essence of a holistic medical practice.

The human body is wonderfully designed. We were created to have good health through old age. A healthy immune system should be able to distinguish between self and non-self. When confronted with a foreign invader, whether it be viral, bacterial, parasitic, or fungal, a healthy immune system should be able to neutralize and destroy any pathogenic organism. In fact, since the beginning of time, the immune system has had to adapt and learn how to overcome pathogenic organisms, or the human race would not have survived.

In the case of viral illnesses, our immune system, when given the basic raw materials it needs, should be able to respond appropriately by neutralizing and removing the virus from the circulation. An unhealthy immune system, however, will struggle with that task.

Americans have been unhealthy for decades. This should not be news to anyone. Just go out and find a crowd and look at the size of the average American. Two-thirds of Americans are overweight, and one-third is obese. We suffer from far too many chronic illnesses, including diabetes, cancer, hypertension, heart disease, and autoimmune disorders. When compared to other Western countries, in nearly every category used to measure the health of a society—such as infant mortality, maternal mortality, chronic illness, and longevity—Americans finish last, or next to last *in every single category!* This is a tragedy and should be unacceptable.

Yet, here we are.

We do not have to continue along this unhealthy road. In my 28 years of experience in seeing patients, I can state, with authority, that things can change. I have seen many unhealthy patients change their trajectory, overcome disease, and improve their health. This is what motivates me in medicine: empowering a patient, through knowledge, about how to achieve their optimal health.

How do you find a healthier road? Adopting some simple changes can start the ball rolling. Eating a healthy diet and avoiding refined food sources, including food with refined sugar, is a start. Maintaining good hydration is a must. Correcting nutrient and hormonal imbalances has proven to help many patients achieve their optimal health. There are many things you can do to not only improve your health but also aid your immune system so that it can do its job of protecting you. I have written fifteen books (this is number sixteen!) about what works in a holistic medical practice to improve your health and help you have a strong immune system.

This book is being written in the midst of the COVID-19 pandemic. The media and the powers-that-be, including the Centers for Disease Control and Prevention (CDC), Department of Health and Human Services (HHS), Food and Drug Administration (FDA), and the Federal Trade Commission (FTC) have all worked together to not only suppress needed information on how to support the immune system but also to keep you in a perpetual state of fear because they want you to believe that there is only one solution for the COVID-19 pandemic: a vaccine. They tell us there is no cure for COVID-19 until a vaccine is developed. They issue edicts that the only thing we can do is to shelter in place, wear masks, and socially distance until the vaccine is developed.

Well, I can tell you, that is not the whole story. There are many things we can do to help our body overcome any viral infection, including COVID-19. You may be familiar with these viruses and their acronyms: HIV, flu, avian flu, SARS, MERS, SARS-CoV-2, and the Hong Kong Flu. Each of these viruses have been present during my lifetime and the vast majority of us—well over 99%—have survived.

What can you do to help your body fight against a viral illness?

The key to winning the battle against a viral or any other infection is having a strong immune system that can neutralize and remove a pathogenic agent.

Let us look at the COVID-19 statistics as I write this book. As of today's writing, the CDC reports that there are 7,824,485 cases of COVID-19 in the United States. The number of deaths is 217,925. _Recovered_ cases stand at 5,019,001.

How did these people recover? These COVID-19 patients recovered because their immune system appropriately responded and overcame SARS-CoV-2.

Therefore, an immune system that can appropriately respond and neutralize SARS-CoV-2 is the remedy for COVID-19. How can you help your immune system properly deal with and overcome SARS-CoV-2? My observation, based on long experience in clinical practice as well as treating COVID-19 patients, is that supplying the immune system with the basic raw materials it needs can enable the immune system to do its job and protect us in times of viral and other infectious illnesses. This should not be a radical concept. I believe all doctors should be evaluating their patients for the status of their nutrient levels and correcting deficiencies *before* someone becomes ill with a virus or other pathogenic organism.

For 28 years, I (and my practice partners) have witnessed how an immune system can be properly supported to aid its response to viral and other illnesses. In fact, I feel my first 27 years as a practicing physician were ideal preparation for something like the current viral pandemic, where the prevailing assumption is that there is no immunity and no treatment available. When COVID-19 was starting on the West Coast of the US, I had a meeting with my staff. Everybody was on edge at this meeting. I told my staff that, to the best of my knowledge and abilities, I thought that we were going to have positive results in our patients who became ill with SARS-CoV-2. I explained that in our experience, patients with influenza-like illnesses (of which, some were coronaviruses) did not, as a rule, end up hospitalized with pneumonia or die. Our patients received immune support that allowed them to appropriately respond to and overcome these viral illnesses. I predicted the same would be true with SARS-CoV-2. And, so far, it has been successful.

To share this approach, I published a peer-reviewed paper, which can be found in the Appendix. This paper documents the wonderful results my practice partners and I have observed in 107 patients who overcame COVID-19 by taking a combination of nutritional and oxidative therapies that make use of essential, all-natural substances to the human body. This is the same therapeutic approach—with small adjustments as we learned new things—that we have been using for 28 years!

This book will provide you with a pathway to provide your immune system with the raw materials it needs to respond, neutralize, and overcome a pathogenic organism such as a virus like SARS-CoV-2.

I do not make a claim that my treatment program will help everyone all the time. Everyone is a unique biochemical individual who needs individualized treatments. However, I believe every immune system can function better if it has the basic raw materials it needs when it is confronted with a viral or other pathogenic organism.

You do not need to have a medical education to understand these concepts. You just need an inquisitive mind. The concepts I share in this book should be easy to understand if I am doing my job correctly. I have seen positive results play out in my practice and I see no reason why it cannot be done elsewhere. You might not hear this information from the powers-that-be, but you should hear it from your holistic doctor. If you do not have a holistic doctor, it is time to find one. A good place to start is the International College of Integrative Medicine (www.icimed.com) where I am a member and on the board of directors.

COVID-19 should be a wakeup call for Americans. The carnage it has caused and is causing did not have to occur. Moving forward, let us make sure nothing like this happens again. You can rest assured that other viruses will be around in the future. The way to combat these pathogens resides within us—a strong, well-supported immune system.

Chapter 2

The Innate and Adaptive Immune Systems

The Innate and Adaptive Immune Systems

Sheila is a 58-year-old hair stylist who became ill with cold and flu-like symptoms. "At first, I thought it was just a cold. But then came the cough, which did not stop. Then the fevers came. They would fluctuate between 100° and 103°[F]. As each day went on, I became weaker and weaker," she said. After eight days of feeling more and more ill, Sheila asked her brother to take her to the emergency room. "I really did not want to go to the hospital. It was right in the middle of COVID-19 and I was scared that I was going to die," she stated.

Sheila was admitted for having difficulty breathing as her pulse oximetry rate was low at 88% [normal is 92-99%]. In the emergency room, Sheila was diagnosed with bilateral pneumonia and started on antibiotics and oxygen therapy. Sheila was placed in a COVID-19 room and isolated. For the first three days of her hospital stay Sheila was given antibiotics, but they were stopped on day four. Sheila stated: "The doctor came in and told me that my test was positive for coronavirus and that I was suffering from COVID-19. He said the pneumonia was viral and that I did not need antibiotics. That was the last time I saw a doctor. The next three days went on and I received no therapy except for oxygen. On day seven, I asked to be sent home as I had to get out of there. They were literally doing nothing for me. Although I was still having breathing issues, I thought I would be more comfortable at home. And, I wanted to call Dr. B."

When Sheila called me, I had a hard time hearing her, as she sounded out of breath. I advised Sheila to start oral vitamins—A, C, D and iodine along with nebulizing hydrogen peroxide. Within a few hours of starting the regimen, Sheila improved. "I could not believe the results. I spent over a week in the hospital and felt terrible. I took your supplements and started nebulizing. Two hours later, I was much better. I don't understand how this therapy is not being done in the hospitals," she said.

Sheila's case is not unique. At my office, we have, as of this writing, treated 120 COVID-19 patients. All our COVID-19 patients have improved, and most experienced symptomatic improvement within a few hours of starting the regimen. The entire regimen was designed to support the immune system and allow the body to overcome a pathogenic organism.

Introduction

The only way to cure oneself from a pathogenic organism, whether it be a virus, bacteria, parasite, retrovirus, fungi, yeast or mold, is for the immune system to react, destroy, and remove the offending organism. Big Pharma would like us to believe that drugs can cure infections. That is not true. Antibiotic, antiviral, anti-parasitic, and anti-fungal medications help by lowering the burden of the infectious organism, but in the end, it is the immune system's responsibility to not only rid the body of a foreign invader, but to provide long-term immunity in order for the body to neutralize the invader if it comes back in the future.

In this book, I will show you how 107 patients were successfully treated for COVID-19 with a treatment program that was designed to provide the immune system with the proper nutrients in order to optimally function against an influenza-like pathogen. I have published a peer-reviewed paper on this. The paper can be found in the Appendix. As previously mentioned, this program has been used for over 20 years and was developed to treat viral infections during flu season. When COVID-19 roared into town, my practice partners and I were confident that our therapy would aid our patients.

To understand how this program works, it is helpful to have a working knowledge of the two major parts of the immune system:

the innate and adaptive branches. Let me explain this concept to you.

The innate immune system is always on guard and responds first to foreign invaders. It does not depend on antibody production. The innate immune system responds by sending specialized white blood cells to inflamed areas to engulf, or "phagocytize" a foreign pathogen, and then destroy it.

The adaptive branch of the immune system responds after the innate side. It is responsible for activating certain cells known as T and B cells, which produce antibodies and other immune system molecules when a pathogen is detected. The adaptive immune system can differentiate whether an infectious agent is new to the body or one that the body has already seen.

Let us examine each immune system branch in a little more detail.

Innate Immune System

The innate immune system is the first line of response of the body to any foreign invader. This branch of the immune system responds nearly the same way every time it detects a pathogenic substance. It does not provide lifelong immunity and it does not differentiate its response. (Note: I am simplifying a very complex system here.) The innate immune system does not produce antibodies or other substances that neutralize specific pathogens that it has seen before.

The innate immune system consists of:

- White blood cells including specialized white blood cells that remove toxic substances and foreign pathogens

- Chemical mediators called cytokines, which recruit white blood cells and other molecules to inflamed/infected areas of the body.

- The physical barriers to infectious organisms that inhibit their ability to enter the body. The gut lining is an example of this.

White Blood Cells and Innate Immunity

White blood cells circulate in the bloodstream. They are responsible for keeping the bloodstream free of foreign substances and pathogenic organisms. Many of them are phagocytic cells.

Phagocytes

Phagocytes engulf and destroy harmful pathogens and foreign substances. They are quite common in the bloodstream. They are also found in the skin and on mucous membranes. They are found at all points-of-entry into the body and can act quickly if a foreign invader such as a virus presents itself. 'Phagocytes' is a generic term, as there are multiple white blood cells that fall under the category of phagocytes, including neutrophils, monocytes, macrophages, dendritic cells and mast cells.

The white blood cells that make up the innate immune system include:

- Macrophages
- Monocytes
- Neutrophils
- Dendritic cells

Macrophages

Macrophages are large phagocytic cells that circulate in the bloodstream and can be found at specific sites of infection in the body. They are derived from monocytes. Macrophages become very mobile in response to inflammation. They can directly kill viruses and other pathogenic organisms and can also stimulate the adaptive immune system by presenting antigens from foreign substances to T and B cells so that antibodies and other adaptive immune system molecules can be manufactured.

Neutrophils

Also known as polymorphonuclear neutrophils (PMNs), these are the most abundant white blood cells. They are the first responders of host defense against infectious organisms. They migrate to areas of inflammation and infection to kill pathogenic organisms.

Dendritic Cells

Dendritic cells are present where the tissues of the body meet the external world, so they are abundantly found in skin and mucous membranes. Dendritic cells function as a bridge between the innate and adaptive immune system branches. They present antigens to the adaptive immune system T cells. An antigen is a toxin or other foreign substance that induces a response from the immune system such as the production of antibodies. A protein on a virus can function as an antigen. Dendritic cells also produce type 1 interferon, which can stimulate innate white blood cells like macrophages to begin the job of phagocytosis.

Adaptive Immune System

The adaptive immune system, in contrast to the innate immune system, uses immunologic memory to activate a response to a foreign pathogen. When activated, the adaptive immune system releases antibodies and other molecules to identify and destroy pathogenic organisms. The adaptive response takes more time than the innate response.

The cells that are activated in the adaptive branch of the immune system are the T and B cells. These are lymphocytes derived from bone marrow stem cells.

B Cells

B cells circulate initially in the lymph system. When they encounter an antigen, B cells bind the antigen and begin to mature. They can produce antibodies specific for a virus or bacteria. These antibodies can help neutralize a pathogenic organism.

T Cells

Once released from the bone marrow, T cells migrate to the thymus gland. The thymus gland resides under the breastbone. T cells spend time in the thymus maturing into different T cells known as CD4 or CD8 T cells.

T cells do not produce antibodies, rather they can bind to an antigen from a pathogenic virus or a foreign substance. Once bound, they release chemicals to stimulate the B cells and the innate immune system to become active and aid in the neutralization and removal of a pathogen or a foreign substance. CD8+ T cells are a specific part of the adaptive immune system and can target infectious organisms as well as kill virally infected cells.

Both B and T cells can have immunologic memory. That means after an initial response to a specific pathogen, subsequent responses can come quickly as the B and T cells have already been primed by prior exposure.

Adaptive Immune System: Humoral and Cell-mediated Immunity

Humoral and cell-mediated immunity are important components of the adaptive immune response. This is a complex topic that I will explain. Humoral immunity refers to the B cells producing antibodies specific to a pathogen. Cell-mediated immunity is the immune response that does not require antibody production. Cell-mediated immunity is governed by the T cells, which release cytokines and other chemicals when confronted with a foreign antigen. These chemicals can recruit other cytotoxic T cells as well as other innate cells to up-regulate the immune system.

Cytokine Storm and the Immune System

Since the COVID-19 pandemic, we frequently hear the term 'cytokine storm'. Cytokines are tiny proteins secreted by cells of the immune system and have a direct effect on other cells. In other words, cells can communicate with other cells through producing and secreting cytokines. Cytokines can respond locally—to cells nearby—or be released into the bloodstream and affect cells and organs distal to their origin. Once released, cytokines bind to immune cells as well as other cells by attaching to specific receptor sites. Once bound, the target cell is stimulated by the cytokines to respond by releasing other proteins that can have anti-inflammatory or pro-inflammatory actions.

For example, in SARS-CoV-2 infections, increased amounts of pro-inflammatory cytokines such as Il-6 (interleukin 6), and IFN-γ (interferon gamma) are also produced.[1] Many other pro-inflammatory cytokines are produced. Once the pro-inflammatory cytokines are produced it can lead to a dangerous situation, as too much inflammation can lead to many health problems due to an overload of oxidative stress. Severe acute respiratory syndrome (SARS) is an example of a serious health issue many COVID-19 patients have had to overcome. As more inflammatory molecules are released in the lung tissue, it can lead to fluid release from cells, causing edema in the lung tissue. This can result in severe shortness of breath and an inability to properly oxygenate the lungs due to excess fluid in the lung tissue.

Final Thoughts

To be functioning at its highest level, we need both the innate and adaptive immune systems working together. The innate immune system is generally the first branch to respond to a pathogen. The adaptive branch responds by producing antibodies and other substances to fight an infectious agent. The adaptive immune system can provide lifelong immunity through antibodies and other molecules. As you will see, providing the right nutrients can aid the various branches of the immune system to function optimally. Eating healthy food, drinking adequate amounts of water, and exercising daily all help the immune system. Adopting a holistic lifestyle can help both your adaptive and innate immune systems. A healthy immune system, compared to a compromised one, can better neutralize and overcome a viral or other pathogenic organism.

[1] Huang C, Wang Y, Li X, et al. Clinical features of patients infected with 2019 novel coronavirus in Wuhan, China [published correction appears in Lancet. 2020 Jan 30;:]. *Lancet*. 2020;395(10223):497-506. doi:10.1016/S0140-6736(20)30183-5

Chapter 3

Vitamin A

Vitamin A

Jeff (not his real name) is a 46-year-old executive who became ill with COVID-19 in the middle of the pandemic. Over the course of a week, his condition worsened, and he began having difficulty breathing. Jeff spoke with his physician, who told him that there was not much to do and advised him not to go to the emergency room unless he was dying, as the medical therapies offered at that time were not proving to be helpful. Jeff had isolated himself in his house and became so weak he was having trouble getting out of bed.

"I felt like I was going to die. I was scared to go to the emergency room, as all the beds were full. I was watching the news and I did not know what to do. My doctor told me to stay at home unless I could not stand it anymore," he said.

Jeff's neighbor and friend was a patient of Dr. Richard Ng, one of the partners in my medical practice. Jeff's friend told him that he had also been sick with COVID-19 and Dr. Ng had prescribed nebulized hydrogen peroxide and oral supplements.

"At this point, I was willing to do anything. I asked him to bring the items to my house," he said. Jeff began taking the oral protocol of vitamins A, C, D, and iodine along with nebulizing hydrogen peroxide and iodine. "It was like a miracle. I truly felt like I was going to die. As soon as I started the regimen, I began to feel *better. My energy began to come back, and I no longer felt like I was going to die. It only took a few days, but I made a full recovery. I can't understand why every emergency room and hospital is not doing this therapy,"* he stated.

Jeff's story is similar to what many of my patients experienced. I have received many letters and messages from patients and non-patients who passed along my protocol and described how it helped others. I interviewed Jeff for my blog site and posted his story. It was viewed over a million times around the world. Jeff's story needs to be viewed by everybody so that they understand that there is hope in a viral pandemic situation.

Introduction

Vitamin A consists of a group of retinoid compounds that have a wide range of physiological effects including supporting immune system functioning. It is a fat-soluble vitamin. Vitamin A is best known for its important role in vision, but it also affects many other areas of the body, including the immune system, reproductive tissues, and cellular communication. Furthermore, vitamin A is one of the most important nutrients for maintaining the normal function and maintenance of the heart, lungs, kidneys, and other organs. Vitamin A deficiency is a worldwide problem affecting 250 million preschool children and half of all countries.[1]

In children, vitamin A supplementation has been shown to dramatically decrease the mortality from the viral illness measles, as well as diarrheal infections.[2]

History of Vitamin A

For millennia, diseases resulting from vitamin deficiencies were attributed to unknown infectious agents or toxicities. Night blindness is a common sign of vitamin A deficiency and still occurs in underdeveloped countries (more about that later). Ulceration of the cornea of the eye, related to dietary factors, was first reported in 1817 by Magendie. He reported this observation in dogs fed for several weeks on a diet limited to sugar and water. Magendie thought the corneal ulcers were from a deficiency of protein in the diet.

During World War I, a physician conducted a controlled trial of different diets in malnourished Danish children. A diet that consisted of whole milk, butter, and cod liver oil was found to protect against corneal ulcers and night blindness caused by a condition called xeropthalmia. It was hypothesized that a fat-soluble substance present in these foods cured the illness. In 1913, McCollum and Davis discovered a fat-soluble accessory food factor (called fat-soluble A). In 1922, McCollum identified and named the fat-soluble substance vitamin A. In 1925, Fridericia and Holm linked vitamin A deficiency to night blindness in rats.

I find the history of vitamins fascinating. Over 100 years ago, studies of vitamin A—before its chemical structure had even been elucidated—pointed to its important role in immune system functioning. Butterfat, a good source of vitamin A, improved the outcome of infections in malnourished animals and humans.[3] Rats were shown to be more susceptible to infections when they were vitamin A deficient.[4]

Infections and Vitamin A Deficiency

Vitamin A plays an important role in supporting the immune system responses to infectious agents. In fact, vitamin A has been shown to help regulate and support the innate as well as the adaptive immune system. This includes cell mediated immunity (T-cells) and the humoral antibody response (B-cells). [5] [6] The immune system functions best when all facets of the immune system are working in harmony with each other. Adequate vitamin A levels allow this to occur.

Both animal and human research studies have shown that an optimized immune system is dependent on adequate vitamin A levels being present. Animal studies have shown that vitamin A deficiency is associated with a lowered antibody response to a variety of vaccines, including tetanus toxoid, rotavirus, diphtheria, pertussis, *Escherichia coli* and bacterial polysaccharide antigens.[7]

Multiple aspects of the immune system are affected by vitamin A deficiency, which causes impaired cell-mediated immunity, decreased proliferation of lymphocytes (which are important in viral infections), decreased natural killer cell activity, and lowered interferon production.[8][9].

Vitamin A is fundamental in maintaining the integrity of the epithelium.[10] Vitamin A deficiency has been associated with disruptions in normal epithelium of the respiratory tract[11][12] and gastrointestinal tissue.[13][14] This disruption can lead to an easier entry point for viral or other pathogens.

Vitamin A deficiency is also associated with problems involving mucosal membrane permeability. Viruses frequently gain entry into the body through the oral or nasal cavities. When the lining of these cavities—the mucosal membrane—is disrupted, it allows an easier entry for a viral (or bacterial) agent. One process that protects this lining is the production of mucus. Mucus is produced from goblet cells, which are found in the epithelial lining (outer tissue layer) of organs such as the intestinal and respiratory tracts. Goblet cells are found inside the trachea, bronchi, and larger bronchioles of the respiratory tract, as well as in the small and large intestines and the conjunctiva in the upper eyelid. A loss of goblet cells has been observed in vitamin A deficiency, and goblet cells have been shown to repopulate tissue with vitamin A supplementation.[15] Vitamin A has also been shown to be an important regulator of monocyte (a white blood cell which helps fight infections) differentiation and function.[16]

Vitamin A and Inflammation

A deficiency of vitamin A can lead to an inflammatory condition. One study compared vitamin A deficient, non-colitic rats to vitamin A sufficient rats. The vitamin A deficient rats had multiple inflammatory signs in their colon consisting of infiltration of inflammatory cells, fibrosis, and activation of nuclear factor kappa β. Vitamin A supplementation ameliorated the infiltration of inflammatory cells in the rats.[17] An inverse relationship between vitamin A levels and inflammation has been reported in other studies.[18] [19]

Acute and chronic inflammation increase vitamin A needs by various tissues and organs of the body, and can result in vitamin A deficiency.[20] Vitamin A has been reported to be helpful in many different inflammatory conditions including inflammatory problems in the lungs, skin, gastrointestinal tract, and in various infectious diseases, including those that can lead to pneumonia.[21] This same study found vitamin A supplementation reduced the severity of childhood pneumonia in developing countries.

My experience with using vitamin A in pneumonia patients (or in those with any upper respiratory symptoms) has been clear: vitamin A supplementation is safe and effective at helping patients recover uneventfully from viral and bacterial upper respiratory and pneumonia infections.

Vitamin A and the Respiratory Tract

Vitamin A is essential for the normal functioning and development of the respiratory tract. Like the gastrointestinal tract, vitamin A deficiency leads to the replacement of the normal ciliated respiratory epithelium (the outer coating of the bronchi) with squamous epithelium.[22] This impairs the ability of the hair-like cilia that line the respiratory tract to remove foreign pathogens. Researchers have reported that mild vitamin A deficiency results in altered pathology of the respiratory tract, which increases the risk for respiratory infections.[23] Low vitamin A levels have been associated with children ill with respiratory syncytial virus (RSV), and low levels of vitamin A are furthermore associated with severe RSV illness.[24]

Vitamin A deficiency in rats has been associated with emphysematous lungs in rats.[25] Lung proinflammatory molecules TNF-α and nitric oxide were found to be elevated in vitamin A deficiency.[26] Human studies have correlated vitamin A deficiency with chronic obstructive lung disease and altered pulmonary function tests.[27] High vitamin A levels and a higher vitamin A intake have been associated with a lower prevalence of shortness of breath in patients with chronic obstructive lung disease.[28]

Researchers who studied a rat asthma model, where the rats developed bronchoconstriction, found a depletion of liver vitamin A stores and increased inflammation in the lungs. The authors concluded, "We postulate that supplementation with vitamin A during airway bronchoconstriction may have some potential benefit by accelerating bronchial epithelial repair following asthmatic attacks, and consequently may reduce the sensitivity of the respiratory mucosa against inflammatory attacks."[29] I have no doubt that this same effect of reducing the sensitivity of the respiratory mucosa against inflammatory attacks and the repair of the bronchial lining would help a patient suffering from lung issues due to a viral illness.

Vitamin A and Mortality

It is well established that vitamin A deficiency can lead to an increase in mortality during times of infection. This was illustrated over 100 years ago in children who were found to have a high mortality rate from many different illnesses including infectious illnesses when they had xeropthalmia. This is the destructive dry-eye condition mentioned earlier in this chapter. It results from vitamin A deficiency causing the epithelia (outer layer) of the cornea of the eyes to become very dry, and can lead to blindness.

The first sign of xeropthalmia due to vitamin A deficiency is often night blindness. It was described in an ancient Egyptian medical treatise dated from between 1520 and 1600 BCE, which recommended eating ox liver or liver of black cocks to cure it.[30] The liver is the body's major storage site for vitamin A. Therefore, in cases of vitamin A deficiency, liver can be an appropriate food source.

Xeropthalmia is still a common problem in developing countries. In fact, night blindness xeropthalmia due to vitamin A deficiency can be cured with vitamin A supplements.

Food Sources and Recommended Intakes of Vitamin A

Vitamin A is found in animal food sources including dairy products, fish, meat and organs, especially the liver, where the majority of the body's vitamin A is stored. The Recommended Daily Allowance (RDA) for a nutrient is the average daily level of intake sufficient to meet the nutrient requirements of nearly all (97-98%) healthy individuals. The RDA for vitamin A in men is 900 µg and in women is 700 µg per day. Table 1 shows vitamin A levels in selected food sources.[31] It is important to note that the highest content of vitamin A in a food source is in liver. If you are going to use liver as a way to ensure adequate vitamin A levels, it is best to use an animal source where the animal is fed a healthy diet free of pesticides, insecticides, herbicides, and synthetic hormones.

Table 1: Selected Food Sources of Vitamin A[32]

Food	Micrograms (mcg) RAE per serving	Percent DV*
Beef liver, pan fried, 3 ounces	6,582	731
Sweet potato, baked in skin, 1 whole	1,403	156
Spinach, frozen, boiled, ½ cup	573	64
Pumpkin pie, commercially prepared, 1 piece	488	54
Carrots, raw, ½ cup	459	51
Ice cream, French vanilla, soft serve, 1 cup	278	31
Cheese, ricotta, part skim, 1 cup	263	29
Herring, Atlantic, pickled, 3 ounces	219	24
Milk, fat free or skim, with added vitamin A and vitamin D, 1 cup	149	17

Table 1: Selected Food Sources of Vitamin A[32]

Food	Micrograms (mcg) RAE per serving	Percent DV*
Cantaloupe, raw, ½ cup	135	15
Peppers, sweet, red, raw, ½ cup	117	13
Mangos, raw, 1 whole	112	12
Breakfast cereals, fortified with 10% of the DV for vitamin A, 1 serving	90	10
Egg, hard boiled, 1 large	75	8
Black-eyed peas (cowpeas), boiled, 1 cup	66	7
Apricots, dried, sulfured, 10 halves	63	7
Broccoli, boiled, ½ cup	60	7
Salmon, sockeye, cooked, 3 ounces	59	7

Table 1: Selected Food Sources of Vitamin A[32]

Food	Micrograms (mcg) RAE per serving	Percent DV*
Tomato juice, canned, ¾ cup	42	5
Yogurt, plain, low fat, 1 cup	32	4
Tuna, light, canned in oil, drained solids, 3 ounces	20	2
Baked beans, canned, plain or vegetarian, 1 cup	13	1
Summer squash, all varieties, boiled, ½ cup	10	1
Chicken, breast meat and skin, roasted, ½ breast	5	1
Pistachio nuts, dry roasted, 1 ounce	4	0

The National Health and Nutrition Examination Survey (2007-2008) reported that the average intake of vitamin A for both men and women in the United States falls below the RDA for vitamin A.[33]

The absorption of vitamin A from the diet, like other fat-soluble vitamins, depends on the body's ability to absorb and metabolize dietary fat. Diseases that cause problems with fat digestion such as Crohn's disease, celiac disease, pancreatic illnesses and hypochlorhydria can negatively affect vitamin A absorption and transport in the body. Since nearly all of the body's vitamin A is found in the liver, when the liver's store of vitamin A becomes depleted, blood serum levels will fall.

What About Beta Carotene?

Carotenoids refer to a diverse group of fat-soluble compounds found in red and yellow-pigmented plant products. Humans consume approximately 40-50 of these carotenoids, primarily in fruits and vegetables.[34] Smaller amounts of carotenoids are found in poultry, egg yolks and seafood.[35] Examples of commonly ingested carotenoids include beta carotene, lutein, and zeaxanthin. Some carotenoids—beta carotene, for example, can be metabolized into vitamin A. However, this process is energy inefficient. Approximately 12 µg of beta carotene are required to produce 1 µg of vitamin A. The conversion of beta carotene into vitamin A is highly variable.

Beta carotene does not provide the body with the immune benefits and anti-pathogenic effects that vitamin A does. For treating a pathogenic condition or supporting the immune system, vitamin A is preferred over beta carotene.

Over 20 years ago I learned that Vitamin A is a therapeutic treatment for influenza-like Illnesses. I read the literature showing how vitamin A helped prevent complications in measles infections. Furthermore, there was a plethora of research showing vitamin A improving the functioning of the innate and adaptive branches of the immune system.

Once I became educated about vitamin A, I began to utilize short-term (four-day), high-dose vitamin A therapy to aid my patients suffering from viral infections.

Vitamin A, in combination with other nutrients such as vitamins C, D, and iodine, were all found to be helpful for those suffering from viral illnesses, particularly in my patients suffering from influenza-like illnesses.

When it became apparent that SARS-CoV-2 was going to cause a pandemic, I felt that vitamin A would aid the immune system in multiple ways to properly respond to the illness. To reemphasize, it is the immune system that ultimately must conquer a pathogenic virus (or bacteria, parasite, etc.,). Antibiotics and antiviral medications along with a targeted vaccine are all suboptimal therapeutic options if the immune system is unable to respond against a pathogenic agent. In my practice, I found vitamin A to be very helpful for COVID-19 patients, just as I have found it useful over the last 20 years for patients suffering from influenza-like as well as other viral illnesses.

Caution with Vitamin A

Vitamin A is a fat-soluble vitamin, as are vitamins D, E, and K. All fat-soluble vitamin supplementation should be undertaken with the advice and monitoring of your doctor. All fat-soluble vitamins can accumulate in the body and therefore become toxic. Hypervitaminosis A is the name of the illness caused by ingesting too much vitamin A. Hypervitaminosis A is associated with increased intracranial pressure (pseudotumor cerebri), dizziness, headaches, nausea, skin irritation, pain in joints and bones, coma, and death. I have not observed toxicity issues (hypervitaminosis A) when prescribing vitamin A for short-term use—four days or less. However, I do not recommend taking vitamin A without your nutritionally-literate doctor following your situation.

Final Thoughts

Vitamin A can be a helpful adjunct to the immune system by allowing it to respond appropriately to a pathogenic infection. As you can see from the discussion in this chapter, vitamin A has multiple positive mechanisms to aid the body in fighting a viral or other infection.

Keep in mind that beta carotene will not provide the same benefits. Emulsified vitamin A is a safer version to take. There is less chance of developing hypervitaminosis A with this source of vitamin A versus vitamin A from fish liver. However, in a pinch, if you are ill, vitamin A from fish liver, over a short time period, can be safely taken.

[1] Who.int. 2020. *WHO | Micronutrient Deficiencies*. [online] Available at: <https://www.who.int/nutrition/topics/vad/en/> [Accessed 7 June 2020].

[2] Eduardo Villamor, Wafaie W. Fawzi, Vitamin A Supplementation: Implications for Morbidity and Mortality in Children, *The Journal of Infectious Diseases*, Volume 182, Issue Supplement_1, September 2000, Pages S122–S133, https://doi.org/10.1086/315921

[3] Osborne TB, Mendel LB, Ferry EL, Wakeman AJ. THE RELATION OF GROWTH TO THE CHEMICAL CONSTITUENTS OF THE DIET. *Journal of Biological Chemistry*. 1913;15:311-326.

[4] Green H. N., Mellanby E.. VITAMIN A AS AN ANTI-INFECTIVE AGENT *Br Med J* 1928; 2 :691

[5] Stephensen CB: Vitamin A, infection, and immunity. Annu Rev Nutr 2001;21:167-192

[6] Villamor E, Fawzi WW: Effects of vitamin A supplementation on immune responses and correlation with nutritional outcome. Clin Microbiol Rev 2005;18: 446-464

[7] Semba, RD, Vitamin A, Immunity, and Infection, *Clinical Infectious Diseases*, Volume 19, Issue 3, September 1994, Pages 489–499, https://doi.org/10.1093/clinids/19.3.489

[8] Tracey A. Bowman, I. Michael Goonewardene, Ana Maria G. Pasatiempo, A. Catharine Ross, Jeff E. Taylor, Vitamin A Deficiency Decreases Natural Killer Cell Activity and Interferon Production in Rats, *The Journal of Nutrition*, Volume 120, Issue 10, October 1990, Pages 1264–1273, https://doi.org/10.1093/jn/120.10.1264

[9] Reifen, Ram. Vitamin A as an anti-inflammatory agent. Proceed. of the Nutritional Society. (2002),61;397-400

[10] Villamor E, Fawzi WW. Effects of vitamin a supplementation on immune responses and correlation with clinical outcomes. *Clin Microbiol Rev*. 2005;18(3):446-464. doi:10.1128/CMR.18.3.446-464.2005

[11] Freudenberg, N., Freudenberg, M.A., Guzman, J. *et al*. Identification of endotoxin-positive cells in the rat lung during shock. *Vichows Archiv A Pathol Anat* **404,** 197–211 (1984). https://doi.org/10.1007/BF00704064

[12] Wong YC, Buck RC. An electron microscopic study of metaplasia of the rat tracheal epithelium in vitamin A deficiency. *Lab Invest*. 1971;24(1):55-66.

[13] Wannee Rojanapo, Adrian J. Lamb, James A. Olson, The Prevalence, Metabolism and Migration of Goblet Cells in Rat Intestine following the Induction of Rapid, Synchronous Vitamin A Deficiency, *The Journal of Nutrition*, Volume 110, Issue 1, January 1980, Pages 178–188, https://doi.org/10.1093/jn/110.1.178

[14] Rosemary A. Warden, Marisa J. Strazzari, Peter R. Dunkley, Edward V. O'Loughlin, Vitamin A-Deficient Rats have Only Mild Changes in Jejunal Structure and Function, *The Journal of Nutrition*, Volume 126, Issue 7, July 1996, Pages 1817–1826, https://doi.org/10.1093/jn/126.7.1817

[15] Sommer, A, Green, William. Goblet Cell Response to Vitamin A treatment for Corneal Xerophthalmia. Am. J. of Opthalmology. Vol. 94;2:August 1982.p. 214-215

[16] Dillehay, D., Walia, A. and Lamon, E. (1988), Effects of Retinoids on Macrophage Function and IL-1 Activity. J Leukoc Biol, 44: 353-360. doi:10.1002/jlb.44.5.353

[17] Uni, Z., Zaiger, G., & Reifen, R. (1998). Vitamin A deficiency induces morphometric changes and decreased functionality in chicken small intestine. *British Journal of Nutrition, 80*(4), 401-407. doi:10.1017/S0007114500070008

[18] Sauer, J.M., et al. All-*trans*-Retinol Alteration of 1-Nitronaphthalene-Induced Pulmonary and Hepatic Injury by Modulation of Associated Inflammatory Responses in the Male

Sprague-Dawley Rat. Toxicology and Applied Pharmacology, Volume 133, Issue 1, July 1995, Pages 139-149

[19] Grace P. Swamidas, Randall J. Basaraba, Richard C. Baybutt, Dietary Retinol Inhibits Inflammatory Responses of Rats Treated with Monocrotaline, The Journal of Nutrition, Volume 129, Issue 7, July 1999, Pages 1285–1290, https://doi.org/10.1093/jn/129.7.1285

[20] Biesalski, HK, et al. Biochemical, morphological and functional aspects of systemic and local vitamin A deficiency in the respiratory tract. Annals of the NY Academy of Sciences. 1992. 559;325-331

[21] The Vitamin A and Pneumonia Working Group (1995). Poteintal intervention of the prevention of childhood pneumonia in developing countries: a meta-analysis of data from field trials to assess the impact of vitamin A supplementation on pneumonia morbidity and mortality. Bulletin of the World Health Organization 73;609-619

[22] McDowell, EM et al. Virchows Arch. B Cell Pathol. 45:197-219

[23] Sommer, J Katz, I Tarwotjo, Increased risk of respiratory disease and diarrhea in children with preexisting mild vitamin A deficiency, The American Journal of Clinical Nutrition, Volume 40, Issue 5, November 1984, Pages 1090–1095, https://doi.org/10.1093/ajcn/40.5.1090

[24] Biesalski, HK, et al. Biochemical, morphological and functional aspects of systemic and local vitamin A deficiency in the respiratory tract. Annals of the NY Academy of Sciences. 1992. 559;325-331

[25] Baybutt, RC, et al. Vitamin A deficiency injures lung and liver parenchyma and impairs function of rat type II pneumocytes. Journal of Nutrition. 2000. 130;1159-1165.

[26] Reifen, Ram. IBID. Vitamin A as an anti-inflammatory agent. Proceed. of the Nutritional Society. (2002),61;397-400

[27] Morabia, A, et al. Serum retinal and airway obstruction. Am. J. of Epidem. 1990. 132;77-82.

[28] Rautalahti, Mi, et al. The effect of topical alpha tocopherol and beta carotene supplementation on COPD symptoms. 1997. Am. J. of Resp Critical Care Med. 156;1447-1452

[29] Reifen, Ram. IBID. Vitamin A as an anti-inflammatory agent. Proceed. of the Nutritional Society. (2002),61;397-400

[30] Accessed 6.23.20. https://www.world-medicinehistory.com/2013/06/history-of-xerophthalmia.html

[31] Accessed 6.23.20. https://ods.od.nih.gov/factsheets/VitaminA-HealthProfessional/

[32] IBID: Accessed 6.23.20. https://ods.od.nih.gov/factsheets/VitaminA-HealthProfessional/

[33] U.S. Department of Agriculture, Agricultural Research Service. What We Eat in America, 2007-2008

[34] Accessed 6.24.20 https://www.cdc.gov/nutritionreport/pdf/Fat.pdf

[35] Boylston T et al. Chemical and biochemical aspects of color in muscle foods. In: Perez-Alvarez, JA, and Fernandez-Lopez   J, editors. Handbook of meat, poultry, and seafood quality. Ames (IA): Blackwell   Publishing; 2007. pp. 25–44

Chapter 4

Vitamin C

Vitamin C

Alan and Peggy are married and have been patients of mine for 15 years. Alan called me and said, "Peggy and I are both sick. We have fevers of 101 degrees, chills, aches and pains. We both have a sore throat. I am really worried for Peggy because you know how bad her lungs are."

Peggy has a long history of asthma and difficulty breathing. She gets lung involvement with simple colds. Over the years we have been able to manage most of her symptoms with intravenous vitamin C treatments when she becomes ill. Alan stated, "This time I am really worried. I have been reading those stories about COVID and people dying because their lungs fill up with fluid. Do you think that could happen to Peggy?"

Alan mentioned that he did not want to go to the emergency room because too many people were dying there. I told Alan that the same antiviral program that I have prescribed for Peggy over the past two decades has worked for our COVID-19 patients. *"I can't guarantee you anything,"* I told Alan, *"but our patients are doing well with COVID-19 and I see no reason why Peggy can't improve. Just make sure she is taking the oral protocol of vitamins A, C, D, and iodine. I think you both should come to the office for IVs of vitamin C and hydrogen peroxide, and let's do an intramuscular shot of ozone as well."*

I met both Alan and Peggy in the parking lot, as we were not letting ill COVID-19 patients into our office. Peggy was treated with the IV and intramuscular therapies of vitamin C, hydrogen peroxide and ozone. The next day, I called them to see how they were doing. "It was amazing," Alan said. "On the way home, Peggy started to feel better. Her aches and pains subsided about three hours later. That night, we were both sitting on the couch watching a movie. The cough settled down and the wheezing went away. Thank you so much. I was really worried about this one." He also stated, "It is hard to believe there is such an easy solution out there, and not everyone is taking advantage of it."

Peggy responded to my protocol the exact same way she has responded over the last 15 years when she has been confronted with other viral and bacterial illnesses. COVID-19 is part of the coronavirus family. Over my medical career I have undoubtably treated many patients infected with various coronaviruses even though I did not test for it. That is why I was confident that our patients with COVID-19 would respond just as our patients have responded over the last 28 years to other influenza-like illnesses. I interviewed Alan (I used a different name for this case history) on my website about how they both responded.

Introduction

When you read the old literature on vitamin C therapy in treating viral infections, it is astounding to me that medical schools across the country are not training their future doctors to be knowledgeable about how and when to use vitamin C in a patient suffering from an infectious agent. I went to medical school at Wayne State University School of Medicine from 1985–1989. I learned little about nutrition and extraordinarily little about vitamin C. I can recall learning that vitamin C deficiency caused scurvy and that scurvy was a disease of the past. That was the extent of my medical school knowledge about vitamin C.

In my holistic training, I learned a lot about vitamin C and why it is such an important, essential nutrient.[1] It is essential because we cannot manufacture it in our bodies, and we cannot live without it. If we do not get enough in our diet, we are deficient. My partners and I have been checking vitamin C levels for over 28 years and I can assure you most of the population is deficient in vitamin C.

Vitamin C

Vitamin C, also called ascorbic acid, is a water-soluble substance found in many food sources such as fruits and vegetables. Every tissue and organ in the body needs and requires vitamin C. Vitamin C is needed to produce collagen, which makes up nearly 75% of the skin and is needed to prevent wrinkles and hold the skin together.[2] A deficiency of collagen is seen with wrinkled, weak skin that is prone to bleeding. Vitamin C is required to produce certain neurotransmitters, plays a role in protein metabolism, and is essential for wound healing.

Vitamin C can function as both an antioxidant and an oxidant in the body. In other words, vitamin C can both donate and receive electrons depending on its status. Iodine is another example of a nutrient that can function as both an antioxidant and an oxidant. This dual ability allows vitamin C to keep other important nutrients and molecules in the body in their anti-oxidation state. Vitamin E and glutathione are examples of other important nutrients that work in concert with vitamin C, sharing electrons. The movement of electrons is what stimulates the production of ATP—the energy molecule that drives cell function.

The immune system cannot function optimally if there is a deficiency of vitamin C. In fact, an infectious illness will acutely increase the body's need for vitamin C.

Vitamin C can be taken both orally and by injection. Orally dosed vitamin C maximizes its absorption below 200 mg/day. Higher dosing of vitamin C orally results in falling absorption levels.

Higher blood levels of vitamin C are needed to assist the immune system during an infectious process. As I stated above, vitamin C absorption declines above 200 mg/day oral dosing. However, intravenous dosing of vitamin C can achieve much higher levels compared to oral dosing.[3]

Nearly 100 years of research has shown the efficacy of vitamin C in treating viral and other pathogenic illnesses. One of the great pioneers of vitamin C therapy in treating infectious illness was Frederick Klenner, M.D., (1907-1984). Dr. Klenner obtained his medical degree from Duke University in 1936. In the early 1950s, Dr. Klenner began to experiment with high doses of vitamin C, both orally and intravenously. He meticulously recorded patients' response to vitamin C and reported these results. He authored 28 peer-reviewed papers during his career.

Vitamin C and Poliomyelitis

One of the first viral illnesses Dr. Klenner successfully treated with vitamin C was polio. Polio was considered an incurable disease. He found high intramuscular or intravenous doses of vitamin C (from 1-2,000 mg in babies to 20,000 mg in adults given multiple times per day), as opposed to small doses, cured polio in multiple case reports.[4] Dr. Klenner found large doses of vitamin C cured many viral infectious diseases. These include:

- Chickenpox
- Herpes infections
- Influenza
- Measles
- Mumps
- Rabies
- Viral encephalitis
- Viral hepatitis
- Viral Pneumonia

Large doses of vitamin C therapy were not just beneficial in those suffering with viral illnesses. Vitamin C therapy was also shown to be effective in bacterial and parasitic illnesses such as:

- Amebic dysentery
- Bacillary dysentery
- Diphtheria
- Leprosy
- Malaria
- Pertussis
- Pseudomonas infection
- Rocky Mountain spotted fever
- Staphylococcal infections

- Streptococcal infections
- Tetanus
- Typhoid fever
- Tuberculosis

Dr. Klenner recorded detailed case histories for each of these disorders.[5] Reading these case histories begets the question, "Why are doctors not using vitamin C to treat patients suffering from infectious illnesses?" In 1951, Dr. Klenner, marking his frustration with conventional medicine's failure to implement his treatments, stated: "Many physicians refuse to employ vitamin C in the amounts suggested, simply because it is counter to their fixed ideas of what is reasonable; but it is not against their reason to try some new product being advertised by an alert drug firm."[6] That quote is especially apropos today as I write this chapter during the COVID-19 pandemic.

How Does Vitamin C Prevent Infections? Hydrogen Peroxide Production

There are multiple mechanisms whereby vitamin C can function as an antiviral agent. Linus Pauling, the two-time Nobel Laurate, promoted the use of vitamin C in treating and preventing viral infections, including the common cold. He suggested that high doses of vitamin C can be directly viricidal.[7] In vivo studies found high dose vitamin C in the presence of free copper and/or iron would generate the production of hydrogen peroxide and other free radicals which could have direct viricidal effects.[8] [9] Also, vitamin C has been shown to have viricidal action against the influenza A virus.

In fact, the observation that ascorbic acid could induce the production of hydrogen peroxide was first reported in 1937.[10] Recall that my protocol for treating COVID-19 consisted of using both vitamin C orally and intravenously along with intravenous hydrogen peroxide. *(See Chapter 7 for more information.)*

Vitamin C and the Immune System

Vitamin C is found in high concentrations in cells that populate the innate immune system. These cells include lymphocytes, leukocytes, and macrophages.[11] Vitamin C has been shown to improve the ability of white blood cells, the first line of defense, to seek out and destroy foreign invaders. It also supports lymphocyte maturation and proliferation and stimulates the phagocytotic (engulfing and destroying) effects of leukocytes.[12] [13]

Interferons are proteins produced and released from cells in response to viral infections. They are aptly named for the ability to interfere with viral replication.[14] Interferons have potent antiviral activity and are produced by white blood cells as well as fibroblasts in response to infection. When they bind to cells that are virally infected, interferons inhibit viral RNA and DNA production. Interferons are used in medicine as treatments for viral infections such as hepatitis B.[15]

Researchers have studied mice that are not able to manufacture their own vitamin C. Nasal inoculation of H3N2 influenza virus into vitamin C-deficient mice was found to significantly increase their mortality compared to mice that could manufacture vitamin C.[16] Furthermore, the scientists reported that vitamin C-deficient mice had inadequate production of anti-viral interferons and other cytokines. The authors summarize their findings by stating, "Taken together, vitamin C shows *in vivo* anti-viral immune responses at the early time of infection, especially against influenza virus, through increased production of [interferons]."

It has been known for over 20 years that patients with infectious diseases have low circulating levels of vitamin C.[17] [18] [19] In fact, critically ill patients have been reported to have a scurvy-like condition due to very low and/or undetectable vitamin C levels.[20] The underlying causes of vitamin C depletion include increased utilization, decreased absorption and increased urinary losses.[21]

Vitamin C can prevent mitochondrial injury. The mitochondria are the energy organelles found in most cells. They produce the energy molecule, ATP. Vitamin C has been shown to prevent oxidative damage in the mitochondria.[22] [23] Mitochondrial damage has been reported in multiple viral infections including SARS-CoV-2.[24] Fatigue, which is common during and after viral infections, can be caused by mitochondrial dysfunction.

Vitamin C and Sepsis

Vitamin C has multiple benefits during an infectious process. Sepsis, which refers to a bloodborne infection, is one of the most dangerous infections a patient can encounter. The role of vitamin C in aiding a patient with sepsis includes having the following abilities:[25]

- Antioxidant
- Anti-clotting
- Anti-inflammatory
- Improves immune function
- Improves microcirculation
- Stimulates and supports wound healing
- Stimulates the synthesis of adrenal hormones necessary for circulatory function

Dr. Paul Marik is a professor of medicine and serves as Pulmonary and Critical Care Medicine Division Chief at Eastern Virginia Medical School. In 2016, he reported that he was treating a patient with overwhelming sepsis, and there was no question that the patient was going to die. He happened to be reading an article about the benefits of vitamin C and thiamine in treating sepsis. He said, "At this point, we had nothing to lose." He administered a cocktail of vitamin B1, vitamin C and steroids. Within days, the patient recovered.[26] Dr. Marik developed a protocol for sepsis that includes the intravenous use of vitamin C, thiamine and steroids and published the results in 2017.[27]

On March 30, 2020, a report stated that Dr. Marik was using his protocol to effectively treat ICU-hospitalized COVID-19 patients. He reported saving four patients including an 86-year-old man with heart disease who was hypoxemic.[28]

Vitamin C and COVID-19

COVID-19 originated in China, and the first cases were identified in Wuhan, China in December 2019. Chinese doctors were the first to treat COVID-19. Infected patients presented with upper respiratory symptoms and, in many, progressed to respiratory failure consistent with acute respiratory distress syndrome (ARDS). ARDS is characterized by fluid building up in the small air sacs of the lung—the alveoli. The fluid impairs the lung's ability to oxygenate red blood cells. Therefore, oxygen levels drop in the body as the tissues and organs are not delivered adequate amounts of oxygen.

As more and more patients were dying in China, doctors began trying other therapies to stem the tide. One of the therapies was using large doses of intravenous (IV) vitamin C. Reports from China stated that 50 moderately ill hospitalized COVID-19 patients were treated with 10 grams of intravenous vitamin C (IVC) and severely ill patients were treated with 20 grams of IV vitamin C daily for seven to ten days. None of the patients treated with IVC died and most reduced their hospitalization stay by three to five days. [29] [30] After these findings were reported, the government of Shanghai, China announced a recommendation that all patients with COVID-19 should be treated with high doses of intravenous vitamin C.

How Does Vitamin C Help COVID-19 Patients?

Once you understand the physiology behind vitamin C, you can see why vitamin C was one of the novel therapies chosen to treat COVID-19. The question of how it helps is a complex topic. For the purposes of this book, I will provide a shorthand answer.

COVID-19 patients are characterized by elevated levels of inflammatory markers and oxidative stress such as high-sensitivity C-reactive protein (hsCRP).[31] Vitamin C is known to have antioxidant and anti-inflammatory effects. Erythrocytes (red blood cells) can deliver oxygen to bodily tissues because they carry iron-containing hemoglobin, which both binds and releases oxygen. Oxidative damage to red blood cells can impair the ability to deliver oxygen to tissues.[32] The management and possibly the prevention of oxidative stress in COVID-19 may be addressed with the use of antioxidant therapies. High-dose IV vitamin C was found to have an antioxidant effect for lung epithelial cells.[33] Vitamin C has also been shown to prevent the oxidation of iron from its reduced ferrous state to the oxidized ferric form.[34] In animal studies, intravenous—but not oral—ascorbate has been shown to act as a stimulator for hydrogen peroxide creation in interstitial fluids. Hydrogen peroxide is a potent antimicrobial agent. More about hydrogen peroxide can be found in Chapter 7.

SARS-CoV-2 can infect cells through its unique viroporin proteins. These proteins form channels that facilitate viral replication and proliferation. This results in a release of inflammasomes, which are part of the innate immune system. Inflammasomes are a complex of proteins found in white blood cells (macrophages and neutrophils) which are responsible for the production of inflammation in innate immunity. In other words, inflammasomes lead to the release of inflammatory cytokines. If this process continues to escalate, it can lead to more inflammation, oxidative stress, and cytokine storm. ARDS is a consequence of this highly inflamed situation. In COVID-19, ARDS has been shown to lead to cellular injury, organ failure and death.[35] Early use of strong antioxidants, such as intravenous vitamin C, could provide an antidote for ARDS. That is the mechanism for Dr. Marik's work on sepsis, described above. One author states,

"Neither intravenous nor oral administration of high-dose vitamin C is associated with significant side effects. Therefore, this regimen should be included in the treatment of COVID-19 and used as a preventative measure for susceptible populations such as healthcare workers with higher exposure risks.[36]

How to Maintain Optimal Vitamin C Levels

As described previously, vitamin C is an essential nutrient that cannot be manufactured in the human body. Therefore, we must get enough from our food or supplement our diets with it. Fruits and vegetables are the best sources of vitamin C. Vitamin C is best ingested by eating raw food sources—in other words, not cooked. The process of heating foods destroys vitamin C.[37] Consuming five servings of fruits and vegetables provides approximately 200 mg of vitamin C, which is above the RDA for vitamin C. The RDA for vitamin C is 75 mg/day for women and 90 mg/day for men.

Recall that the RDA was established to determine the minimal amount of a nutrient that is needed to prevent disease. In the case of vitamin C, the RDA of 75 mg/day means that for the majority (98%) of the population, 75 mg of vitamin C per day is the minimum amount of vitamin C necessary to prevent scurvy or scurvy-associated disorders. It does not mean that this is the *optimal* amount of daily vitamin C for the body. What is the optimal amount of vitamin C? This is a difficult question to answer because when you are ill with a viral or other infection, your vitamin C requirements increase, as vitamin C is rapidly used up in times of stress. Therefore, it is best to increase your vitamin C intake at any time of stress including during an infection or when confronted with a stressful situation. At the end of this chapter I will provide you with my recommendations on vitamin C dosing.

Who is at Risk for Vitamin C Deficiency?

Cigarette smokers are at an increased risk of vitamin C deficiency. Studies dating back over 50 years comparing vitamin C levels between smokers and nonsmokers found smokers have lower blood levels of vitamin C.[38] Smokers have also been found to have lower blood and white blood cell vitamin C levels when compared to nonsmokers. And, smokers were also found to have a lower intake of vitamin C.[39] It should be no surprise that during COVID-19, the World Health Organization found cigarette smokers were at an increased risk for severity of disease among hospitalized patients.[40]

Cancer patients undergoing chemotherapy and radiation will have increased vitamin C needs. In fact, any illness that increases inflammation and oxidative stress will increase the body's need for vitamin C.

Anyone suffering from a viral or other infectious illness is also at an increased risk for vitamin C deficiency. It has been well-established that viral illnesses are associated with oxidative stress.[41] Many different viral illnesses have been associated with low vitamin C levels including hepatitis C,[42] herpes,[43] Epstein Barr virus,[44] and influenza virus.[45]

With regards to influenza virus, an *in vitro* study found pharmacologic levels of ascorbic acid—levels achievable through intravenous dosing in live human and animal studies—killed not only isolated influenza viruses but also viruses from normal human bronchial epithelial cells.[46] Lower doses of vitamin C were able to eliminate 90% of the viruses, and higher doses were able to completely block viral replication. Pharmacologic vitamin C levels eliminated viral infectivity with treatment times as short as four hours at early stages of infection. The authors concluded, "Pharmacological ascorbate (vitamin C) as a pro-drug eliminates or kills influenza virus, probably by producing steady-state concentrations of hydrogen peroxide (H_2O_2) in extracellular fluid."

This same author also studied the effects of pharmacologic dosing of vitamin C against influenza viruses *in vivo*.[47] Mice were inoculated intranasally with influenza and treated with vitamin C injections. Compared to mice not treated with vitamin C, mice given vitamin C injections had higher survival, less weight loss, and had lung influenza viral titers reduced by as much as 10 to 100-fold. The treated mice also were found to have little inflammation in their lung tissues compared to controls. Inflammatory cytokines such as IL-1, IL-6, and IFN-alpha levels were lower in vitamin C-treated mice versus controls.

Final Thoughts

I simply cannot understand why the research and science behind vitamin C was not taught to me and is still not being taught in medical schools.

Vitamin C therapy has thousands of research articles verifying its effectiveness for helping the body recover from and avoid problems with oxidative stress. There are hundreds of peer-reviewed studies showing the effectiveness of vitamin C in treating a wide variety of viral illnesses for which conventional medicine has little to offer.

When COVID-19 started, I had no doubt that I would be using vitamin C both orally and intravenously, and I did not doubt that it would be effective at helping my patients recover from and avoid serious complications. After treating well over 100 patients with COVID-19 (between my partners and me), I can state, with authority, that vitamin C therapy should be the standard of care in any viral illness. Every physician should understand that the failure to use vitamin C in serious viral illnesses such as SARS-CoV-2 can result in serious problems, including death.

For my patients, I have been suggesting daily doses of oral vitamin C in the range of 3-5,000 mg/day in the form of ascorbic acid or buffered vitamin C with ascorbic acid in the ingredients. This is the minimal amount that saturates the red and white blood cells. In times of illness or any increased oxidative stress, vitamin C can be taken in doses of 1,000 mg every hour, in the form of ascorbic acid. If loose stools or diarrhea develop, the dose can be lowered.

It is helpful to work with a doctor who has experience with using vitamin C intravenously. If you become ill with a viral infection, the early use of intravenous vitamin C can provide for a speedy recovery.

Holistic doctors should be literate in the use of oral and intravenous vitamin C. This is one of the main reasons why you should have a holistic doctor taking care of you and your family.

[1] Li Y, Schellhorn HE. New developments and novel therapeutic perspectives for vitamin C. J Nutr 2007;137:2171-8

[2] Schellhorn, Li. IBID. 2007

[3] Sebastian, J, eta l. Vitamin C Pharmacokinetics: Implications for Oral and Intravenous Use. Annals of Int. Med. April 6, 2004.Vol. 140, N.7;533-537

[4] Klnner, F. The treatment of poliomyelitis and other virus disease with vitamin C. July, 1949. Southern Medicien and Surgery. 111.7;209-214.

[5] Levy, Thomas. Vitamin C Infectious Diseases and Toxins.2002.

[6] Accessed 7.2.20 from: https://omarchives.org/dr-frederick-klenner-md-massive-doses-of-vitamin-c-and-the-virus-diseases/

[7] Pauling L. The significance of the evidence about ascorbic acid and the common cold. Proc Natl Acad Sci U S A. 1971;68:2678–2681

[8] While LA, Freeman CY, Forrester BD, et al. In vitro effect of ascorbic acid on infectivity of herpesviruses and paramyxoviruses. J Clin Microbiol. 1986;24:527–531.

[9] Klein M. The mechanism of the virucidal action of ascorbic acid. Science. 1945;101:587–589

[10] Lyman, C.H., et al. Journal of Biol. Chem.1937. 118:757

[11] Carr AC. Vitamin C and Immune Function. Nutrients. 2017;9:1211.

[12] Carr AC. Vitamin C and Immune Function. Nutrients. 2017;9:1211

[13] Leibovitz B, Siegel BV. Ascorbic acid and the immune response. Adv Exp Med Biol. 1981;135:1–25

[14] Parkin J, Cohen B (June 2001). "An overview of the immune system". *Lancet*. **357** (9270): 1777–89

[15] Hoofnagle JH, di Biscerglie AM. The treatment of chronic viral hepatitis. N Engl J Med 1997; 336: 347–56.

[16] Kim Y, Kim H, Bae S, et al. Vitamin C is an essential factor on the anti-viral immune response through the production of interferon-alpha/beta at the initial stage of influenza A virus (H3N2) infection. Immune Netw. 2013;13:70–74

[17] Galley,H.F.;Davies,M.J.;Webster,N.R.Ascorbylradicalformationinpatientswithsepsis: Effectofascorbate loading. Free Radic. Biol Med. 1996, 20, 139–143

[18] Borrelli, E.; Roux-Lombard, P.; Grau, G.E.; Giradin, E.; Ricou, B.; Dayer, J.; Suter, P.M. Plasma concentrations of cytokines, their soluble receptors, and antioxidant vitamins can predict the development of multiple organ failure in patients at risk. Crit. Care Med. 1996, 24, 392–397

[19] Evans-Olders, R.; Eintracht, S.; Hoffer, L.J. Metabolic origin of hypovitaminosis C in acutely hospitalized patients. Nutrition 2010, 26, 1070–1074

[20] Carr, A.C.; Rosengrave, P.C.; Bayer, S.; Chambers, S.; Mehrtens, J.; Shaw, G.M. Hypovitaminosis C and vitamin C deficiency in critically ill patients despite recommended enteral and parenteral intakes. Crit Care 2017, 21, 300

[21] Marik, P. Review Hydrocortisone, Ascorbic Acid and Thiamine (HAT Therapy) for the Treatment of Sepsis. Focus on Ascorbic Acid. Nutrients 2018, 10, 1762; doi:10.3390/nu10111762

[22] Sagun, K.C.; Carcamo, J.M.; Golde, D.N. Vitamin C enters mitochondria via facilitative glucose transporter 1 (Glut1) and confers mitochondrial protection against oxidative injury. FASEB J. 2005, 19, 1657–1667

[23] Lowes, D.A.; Webster, N.R.; Galley, H.F. Dehydroascorbic acid as pre-conditioner: Protection from lipopolysaccharide induced mitochondrial damage. FreeRadic. Res. 2010, 44, 283–292

[24] Saleh, J, et al. Mitochondria and Microbiota dysfunction in COVID-19 pathogenesis. Mitochondrion. In press, Journal Pre-proof available June 20,2020. https://doi.org/10.1016/j.mito.2020.06.008

[25] Marik, P. IBID. 2018.

[26] Accessed 7.3.2020 from: https://hopeforhs.org/dr-paul-marik-potential-cure-for-sepsis/

[27] Marik PE, Khangoora V, Rivera R, Hooper MH, Catravas J. Hydrocortisone, Vitamin C, and Thiamine for the Treatment of Severe Sepsis and Septic Shock: A Retrospective Before-After Study. *Chest*. 2017;151(6):1229-1238. doi:10.1016/j.chest.2016.11.036

[28] Press release March 30, 2020. Three U.S. hospitals use IVs of Vitamin C and other low-cost, readily available drugs to cut the death-rate of COVID-19 — without ventilators! Accessed 7.3.2020 from: http://www.medreview.us/wp-content/uploads/2020/03/3.31.20-Treating-Covid-19-in-ICU.pdf

[29] Shanghai new coronavirus disease clinical treatment expert group. Shanghai 2019 coronavirus disease comprehensive treatment expert consensus. Journal of Infect. Diseases. (Network pre-publishing),38, May 2020.

[30] Accessed 7.4.20 from: http://orthomolecular.org/resources/omns/v16n16.shtml

[31] Chen L, Liu HG, Liu W, et al. *Zhonghua Jie He He Hu Xi Za Zhi*. 2020;43(0):E005. doi:10.3760/cma.j.issn.1001-0939.2020.0005

[32] Mohanty, J., Nagababu, E. and Rifkind, J., 2014. Red blood cell oxidative stress impairs oxygen delivery and induces red blood cell aging. *Frontiers in Physiology*, 5.

[33] Erol A. High-dose intravenous vitamin C treatment for COVID-19. doi:10.31219/osf.io/p7ex8.

[34] Lu P, Ma D, Yan C, Gong X, Du M, Shi Y. Structure and mechanism of a eukaryotic transmembrane ascorbate-dependent oxidoreductase. *Proc Natl Acad Sci U S A*. 2014;111(5):1813-1818. doi:10.1073/pnas.1323931111

[35] Medicine in Drug Discovery. 5(2020). 100028

[36] Medicine in Drug Discovery. IBID. 2020.

[37] Weinstein M, Babyn P, Zlotkin S. An orange a day keeps the doctor away: scurvy in the year 2000. *Pediatrics*. 2001;108(3):E55. doi:10.1542/peds.108.3.e55

[38] Omer, Pelletier, Smoking and Vitamin C Levels in Humans, *The American Journal of Clinical Nutrition*, Volume 21, Issue 11, November 1968, Pages 1259–1267, https://doi.org/10.1093/ajcn/21.11.1259

[39] Schectman, G, et al. The Influence of Smoking on Vitamin C Status in Adults. Am. J. of Pub. Health. Vol. 79, n. 2. February, 1989.158-162

[40] Accessed 8.2.20 from: https://www.who.int/news-room/commentaries/detail/smoking-and-covid-19

[41] Mikirova N, Hunninghake R. Effect of high dose vitamin C on Epstein-Barr viral infection. *Med Sci Monit*. 2014;20:725-732. Published 2014 May 3. doi:10.12659/MSM.890423

[42] Jain SK, Pemberton PW, Smith A, et al. Oxidative stress in chronic hepatitis C: not just a feature of late stage disease. J Hepatol. 2002;36(6):805–11

[43] Chen JY, Chang CY, Feng PH, et al. Plasma vitamin C is lower in postherpetic neuralgia patients and administration of vitamin C reduces spontaneous pain but not brush-evoked pain. Clin J Pain. 2009;25(7):562–69.

[44] Mikirova, N, et al. IBID. 2014.

[45] Cheng LL, Liu YY, Li B, Li SY, Ran PX. *Zhonghua Jie He He Hu Xi Za Zhi*. 2012;35(7):520-523.

[46] Cheng, LL, *et al*. IBID. 2012.

[47] Cheng L, Liu Y, Li B, Ye F, Ran P. *Zhonghua Jie He He Hu Xi Za Zhi*. { **Pharmacologic ascorbate treatment of influenza in vivo**}. 2014;37(5):356-359.

Chapter 5

Vitamin D

Vitamin D

Introduction

Vitamin D was one of the first nutrients touted for helping COVID-19 patients. Keep in mind, the flu season generally begins in January and ends in April/May every year. This is the same timeframe that vitamin D levels are at their lowest in the Northern hemisphere. There have been many studies showing that low vitamin D levels correlate with an increased risk of becoming ill with a viral infection and suffering a more serious case of a viral infection. Although correlation does not equal causation, an inverse correlation between low vitamin D levels and increased risk of a viral infection should call for more studies. In the recent coronavirus pandemic, there have been studies finding low vitamin D levels correlated with an increased risk of infection.

Since the beginning of the COVID-19 pandemic, scientists have proposed that there is a potential inverse association between mean levels of vitamin D in various countries and the number of cases and increased mortality caused by COVID-19.[1] In other words, lower vitamin D levels are associated with increased mortality caused by COVID-19. The mean levels of vitamin D for 20 European countries and morbidity and mortality due to SARS-CoV-2 were studied. Lower vitamin D levels correlated with higher levels of infection and mortality. Vitamin D levels were very low in countries with older populations, especially in Spain, Italy, and Switzerland. The elderly are known to be one of the most vulnerable groups of the population to COVID-19 as well as other influenza-like illnesses. A similar association between low vitamin D levels and increased risk of morbidity and mortality due to COVID-19 has been found in the Philippines.[2]

What Does Vitamin D Do in the Body?

I have been checking vitamin D levels for over 25 years. Most of my patients when initially tested have had low levels of vitamin D. Vitamin D is a fat-soluble vitamin that is misnamed. A vitamin is an essential substance that cannot be manufactured in the body; therefore, it needs to be ingested. However, unlike other vitamins, Vitamin D is produced in the body, after ultraviolet light hits the skin. Vitamin D can also be obtained from food and supplements.

Vitamin D, whether produced in the skin, taken as a supplement, or obtained from food, is inactive. Both the liver and the kidney need to chemically alter it to its active form, known as calcitriol.

Vitamin D has many physiological effects in the body. It helps the intestines absorb calcium from the diet and helps the major bone cells—osteoblasts and osteoclasts—maintain optimal bone mineralization and strength. Vitamin D deficiency can lead to weakened bones. The classic disease associated with vitamin D deficiency is rickets. Rickets is an illness characterized by weakened and softened bones. Rickets is caused by extreme vitamin D deficiency. In the US, rickets is still being diagnosed, mostly in malnourished children. In adults, vitamin D deficiency can lead to weakened bones and a diagnosis of osteoporosis. Maintaining adequate vitamin D levels can help avoid degenerative bone diseases like rickets and osteoporosis.

However, vitamin D is not just for the bones. There are vitamin D receptors throughout the body's tissues, including the prostate, breast, lung, skin, lymph nodes, colon, pancreas, adrenal medulla, and brain—especially in the cerebellum and the cerebral cortex, which is the thinking part of the brain.[3] [4] Vitamin D receptors have also been found in the pancreas, white blood cells (monocytes), immune system cells (B cells and T cells), neurons, ovarian cells, pituitary and aortic endothelial cells.[5]

Vitamin D and the Immune System

Vitamin D has been shown to help both the innate and adaptive branches of the immune system in response to infection. White blood cells are part of the innate immune system response to infectious organisms. As described in Chapter 2, the innate immune system is the first line of response to a pathogenic organism. It responds to a pathogen the same way, each time. It does not provide long-term immunity. Long-term immunity comes from the adaptive immune system.

When confronted with an infectious organism, the monocytes—which evolve into macrophages—respond by engulfing and destroying viruses or bacterial particles. They are also responsible for signaling T cells, the adaptive cells of the immune system, to aid in identifying and removing foreign invaders from the body.[6] Vitamin D is a key link in the ability of the monocyte/macrophage to appropriately respond to infection.[7]

Since vitamin D receptors have been found in so many different tissues of the body, it should be no surprise that vitamin D is such an integral substance, with a wide range of physical effects. Vitamin D has been shown to have immunoregulatory effects as it can lower inflammatory cytokines.[8] Cytokines are inflammatory-producing molecules such as interferon, secreted by immune system cells. (Note: There are other cytokines that stimulate the growth and differentiation of cells.) COVID-19 was characterized by cytokine storm in extremely ill patients, and this inflammatory condition was hypothesized to be a major cause of multi-organ failure, blood clots and death.[9]

Vitamin D Deficiency and Inflammatory Diseases

In over two decades of checking and evaluating vitamin D levels, I can state, with confidence, that lowered vitamin D levels are common in inflammatory illnesses such as severe viral infections, autoimmune disorders, cancer, and other degenerative conditions. Vitamin D is thought to have an anti-inflammatory effect in many chronic illnesses. In fact, studies have shown that vitamin D supplementation can lower commonly measured inflammatory markers such as IL-6 and C-reactive protein (CRP) in critically ill ICU patients.[10]

Chronic obstructive pulmonary disease (COPD) is a chronic, inflammatory lung disease that causes obstruction of the airflow in the lungs. Symptoms of COPD include coughing, mucous production, difficulty breathing, and wheezing. It is the third leading cause of death in the world.[11] COPD is caused by cigarette smoking and other lung irritants. Patients with COPD are more susceptible to viral and bacterial lung infections. Researchers found that patients low in vitamin D_3 (<20 ng/ml) had a 45% reduction in COPD exacerbations when they were supplemented with vitamin D.

Vitamin D and Respiratory Tract Infections

There is a plethora of research indicating that vitamin D can help protect against respiratory illnesses. Researchers assessed the overall effectiveness of vitamin D supplementation on the risk of respiratory tract infections. This was a randomized, double-blind, placebo-controlled trial of supplementation with vitamin D. The scientists reported a 12% decreased risk of acute respiratory infection with vitamin D supplementation. The best results were achieved in those who had severely low vitamin D levels (<10 ng/ml). The authors concluded, "Vitamin D supplementation was safe, and it protected against acute respiratory tract infection overall." [12]

Coronavirus and Vitamin D

Near the beginning of the coronavirus pandemic, there was speculation that lowered vitamin D levels may be a factor in the severity of the illness. Scientists attempted to examine the effect of different vitamin D levels and the severity of COVID-19 in a retrospective study of a cohort of patients from Switzerland.[13] The authors found significantly lower vitamin D levels in laboratory confirmed – Polymerase chain receptor (PCR)-positive– SARS-CoV-2 patients compared with PCR-negative patients. The authors concluded the study by stating: "On the basis of this preliminary observation, vitamin D supplementation might be a useful measure to reduce the risk of infection."

The first randomized, controlled trial of vitamin D and COVID-19 was published as I was finishing this book.[14] The results were astonishing. Scientists from Spain studied 76 consecutive patients hospitalized with COVID-19 who suffered with a clinical picture of acute respiratory infection and pneumonia. All patients received standard care per hospital protocol and a combination of hydroxychloroquine and azithromycin. The patients were randomized to receive vitamin D or no vitamin D. The vitamin D dose used in this study was similar to my four-day dosing regimen of 100,000 IU/day of vitamin D3. In this study, subjects treated with vitamin D were dosed on Day 1 of admission with 106,400 IU and 53,200 IU on days 3 and 7. Of those treated with vitamin D, none died and all were discharged without complications. Fifty percent of the control group (not treated with vitamin D) required admission to the ICU while only 2% of these in the vitamin D group were admitted to the ICU. In other words, compared to those treated with Vitamin D, there was a 25x increase risk in being admitted to the ICU in those not treated with vitamin D. This was a small study, but the results are compelling .

Why Is COVID-19 More Deadly to Minorities?

Coronavirus has affected minorities more severely. According to the CDC, blacks and whites were found to have an age-adjusted hospitalization rate of 178.1 and 40.1 per 100,000 population, respectively.[15] That means black people are hospitalized with coronavirus at a rate approximately *five times* white people are.

Researchers have theorized why this discrepancy exists. Scientists have pointed out that there is less access to health care by minorities, which can limit diagnosis and treatment, leading to poor health outcomes. It is well known that COVID-19 is more problematic when co-morbidities such as hypertension, obesity, asthma, and diabetes are present. Compared to Caucasians, African Americans disproportionly suffer from these comorbidities. Perhaps it is the co-morbidities that are fueling the increased rate of adverse outcomes for African Americans.

There are other socioeconomic reasons such as poverty and cigarette smoking that may explain why minorities may be suffering more adverse outcomes from COVID-19. However, vitamin D status may also provide clues.

Lowered vitamin D levels may be a factor in the racial divide with respect to COVID-19 as well as other viral infections. It has been well known for decades that vitamin D insufficiency is more prevalent among African Americans than other Americans. In fact, studies have reported that young healthy African Americans fail to achieve sufficient vitamin D levels at any time of the year. The main factor driving this epidemic is the fact that pigmented skin reduces vitamin D production.[16] In other words, darker skin requires more sunlight to manufacture vitamin D when compared to lighter skin. Therefore, a darker-skinned individual would require more sun exposure to produce a similar amount of vitamin D than a lighter-skinned person. Adequate vitamin D levels have been associated with lower rates of cancer, heart disease, and diabetes, which are all conditions that disproportionately affect African Americans.

Vitamin D, the Immune System, and COVID-19

How would vitamin D reduce the risk of COVID-19? A review published in April 2020, by William Grant, one of the foremost experts on vitamin D, identified two mechanisms:[17]

- By reducing the survival and replication of viruses through vitamin D-stimulated release of cathelicidin

- By lowering the risk of the cytokine storm by reducing production of pro-inflammatory cytokines

Let's look at those two mechanisms a little closer. Vitamin D has been shown to enhance the innate immune system through the "...induction of antimicrobial peptides including human cathelicidin, LL-37, by 1, 25-dihydroxyvitamin D."[18] Cathelicidens are stored in the lysosomes of macrophages and polymorphonuclear leukocytes. Lysosomes are found in many cells and contain enzymes that help break down pathogenic organisms by digesting them. Cathelicidens work against a broad spectrum of pathogenic organisms including bacteria, viruses (both enveloped and nonenveloped), and fungi.[19] SARS-CoV-2, the virus that causes COVID-19, is an enveloped virus which means it has an outer shell that protects the viral genetic material.

There are other pleiotropic benefits of vitamin D that can result in a reduced risk of infection. Vitamin D has been found to reduce the risk of viral infections like the common cold by improving epithelial barriers, helping prevent a virus from entering the body, as well as by enhancing cellular and adaptive immunity.[20]

A large, population-based study found low vitamin D levels are an independent risk factor for COVID-19 infection and hospitalization.[21] In fact, subjects positive for COVID-19 were 50% more likely to have low vitamin D levels–25(OH)D$_3$– in the final analysis. The senior author of this research paper stated that it is important "...to test patients' vitamin D levels and keep them optimal for the overall health as well as for better immune-response to COVID-19."[22]

Vitamin D and Cytokine Storm

'Cytokine storm' refers to a hyperinflammatory condition where the immune system overreacts to a pathogenic agent. As the out-of-control immune system keeps releasing inflammatory molecules, eventually the organs become overwhelmed. The lungs, kidneys and liver can be adversely affected by cytokine storm. Severely ill COVID-19 patients are characterized by damage to the lungs, kidneys, and liver by the over-production of inflammatory molecules. It is accepted that cytokine storm has led to respiratory failure and death in far too many COVID-19 patients. Cytokine storm and mortality with COVID-19 are more common in the elderly.[23] It is also well established that vitamin D levels decrease with age.[24]

Vitamin D has been shown to reduce the production of pro-inflammatory Th1 cytokines such as TNF-α and interferon-γ.[25] Furthermore, vitamin D supplementation has been shown to reduce the expression of pro-inflammatory cytokines and increase the production of anti-inflammatory cytokines by the innate immune system macrophage cells.[26]

Vitamin D and Adaptive Immune Response

The adaptive immune system is also positively influenced by vitamin D. The active form of vitamin D, $1,25(OH)D_3$, suppresses the T helper cell (Th1) by reducing the production of inflammatory cytokines IL-2 and interferon gamma (INF_γ).[27] Furthermore, the active form of vitamin D has been shown to promote the induction of T regulatory cells, which has been shown to modulate the inflammatory response.[28]

In patients with pneumonia, supplementation with vitamin D3 suppresses the production of proinflammatory cytokines (tumor necrosis factor alpha [TNF-α], gamma interferon [IFN-γ], interleukin-6 [IL-6], and inducible nitric oxide synthase [iNOS]. Furthermore, vitamin D supplementation works to increase the expression of genes that promote the production of antioxidant enzymes such as glutathione reductase and the production of antimicrobial peptides (cathelicidin).[29]

Vitamin D as a Treatment in Viral Infections

As I documented in my peer-reviewed article[30] about treating COVID-19, vitamin D is being researched as an effective treatment option for COVID-19 patients. Researchers used 25-hydroxyvitamin D [25(OH)D] levels as a marker to predict clinical outcomes of COVID-19 subjects.[31] Of 212 cases of COVID-19, serum 25(OH)D level was lowest in critical cases and highest in mild cases. The authors reported vitamin D is significantly associated with clinical outcomes. A logistical regression analysis reported that for each standard deviation increase in serum 25(OH)D, the odds of having a mild clinical outcome rather than a severe outcome were approximately 7.94 times (OR=0.126, p<0.001). Interestingly, the odds of having a mild clinical outcome rather than a critical outcome were approximately 19.61 times (OR=0.051, p<0.001). These results suggest that an increase in serum 25(OH)D level in the body could either improve clinical outcomes or mitigate the worst (severe to critical) outcomes, while a decrease in serum 25(OH)D level in the body could worsen the clinical outcomes of COVID-19 patients.

There are additional mechanisms by which vitamin D could reduce the risk of influenza-like infections and death. Viral infections have been shown to disrupt airway epithelial cell junctions.[32] Vitamin D has been shown to maintain tight epithelial junctions and adherens junctions.[33]

Final Thoughts

I have over two decades of experience in testing for vitamin D. During this same time period, I have been supplementing with vitamin D3 in my patients. I have clearly seen the benefits of ensuring adequate vitamin D levels in the body.

The best way to ensure adequate vitamin D levels is to get vitamin D the natural way; expose your skin to sunlight. Unfortunately, the powers-that-be have frightened us about sun exposure. They state that the sun causes skin cancer therefore we need to avoid exposing our skin to the sun. I agree overexposure to the sun can cause skin problems, but humans were designed to produce vitamin D from sun exposure. It is not wise to get sunburned, but I suggest getting enough sun exposure to aid in the production of vitamin D. I encourage my patients to get 30 minutes of sun exposure during months when there is adequate ultraviolet radiation, so that vitamin D can be manufactured in the skin.

Vitamin D supplementation is safe when levels of vitamin D are followed. Vitamin D is a fat-soluble vitamin, so long-term use of it can cause problems. A short-term large dose of vitamin D, as described in my paper—50,000 Units of vitamin D3 per day for four days–is safe to take during an acute viral illness. Not only is it safe, it is effective at providing the immune system with a nutrient that it needs to aid it in overcoming an infectious organism.

For the best results, I suggest working with a holistic doctor who is vitamin D-literate. Avoid taking synthetic sources of vitamin D—ergocalciferol or vitamin D_2. It is not utilized as well as vitamin D3. Most prescription forms of vitamin D utilize the synthetic version.

[1] Ilie, Petre, et al. The role of vitamin D in the prevention of coronavirus disease 2019 infection and mortality

[2] Alipio, Mark, Vitamin D Supplementation Could Possibly Improve Clinical Outcomes of Patients Infected with Coronavirus-2019 (COVID-19) (April 9, 2020). Available at SSRN: https://ssrn.com/abstract=3571484 or http://dx.doi.org/10.2139/ssrn.3571484

[3] Holick MF. Vitamin D: importance in the prevention of cancers, type 1 diabetes, heart disease, and osteoporosis. Am J Clin Nutr. 2004;79(3):362-71

[4] Zehnder D, Bland R, Williams MC, McNinch RW, Howie AJ, Stewart PM, Hewison M. Extrarenal expression of 25-hydroxyvitamin d(3)-1 alpha-hydroxylase. J Clin Endocrinol Metab. 2001;86(2):888-94.

[5] Zittermann A. Vitamin D in preventive medicine: are we ignoring the evidence? Br J Nutr. 2003;89(5):552-72.

[6] Justiz, Angel, et al. Physiology, Immune Response. Treasure Island (FL): StatPearls Publishing; 2020 Jan

[7] Hewison, M. Vitamin D and the intracrinology of innate immunity. Mol. Cell. Endocrin. 2010;321(2):103-111.

[8] Timms PM, Mannan N, Hitman GA, Noonan K, Mills PG, Syndercombe-Court D, Aganna E, Price CP, Boucher BJ. Circulating MMP9, vitamin D and variation in the TIMP-1 response with VDR genotype: mechanisms for inflammatory damage in chronic disorders? QJM. 2002;95:787-96.

[9] Jose, R, et al. The Lancet Respiratory Medicine. Volume 8:6,E46-47, June 1, 2020.

[10] Van den Berghe G, Van Roosbroeck D, Vanhove P, Wouters PJ, De Pourcq L, Bouillon R. Bone turnover in prolonged critical illness: effect of vitamin D. J Clin Endocrinol Metab. 2003;88(10):4623-32.

[11] Terzikhan, N, et al. Prevalence and incidence of COPD in smokers and non-smokers: the Rotterdam Study. Eur. J. of Epidemiology. 2016;31(8):785-792

[12] BMJ 2017; 356 doi: https://doi.org/10.1136/bmj.i6583 (Published 15 February 2017)

[13] D'Voloio, A, et al. 25-Hydroxyvitamin D Concentrations Are Lower in Patients with Positive PCR for SARS-CoV-2. Nutrients. 2020. 12(5):1359; https://doi.org/10.3390/nu12051359

[14] Castillo ME, Entrenas Costa LM, Vaquero Barrios JM, Alcaĺ aD´ıazJF, Miranda JL, Bouillon R, Quesada Gomez JM,"Effect of Calcifediol Treatment and bestAvailable Therapy versus best Available Therapy on Intensive Care Unit Admission andMortality Among Patients Hospitalized for COVID-19: A Pilot Randomized Clinical study",Journal of Steroid Biochemistry and Molecular Biology(2020),doi:https://doi.org/10.1016/j.jsbmb.2020.9

[15] Accessed 6.25.20 from: https://www.cdc.gov/coronavirus/2019-ncov/need-extra-precautions/racial-ethnic-minorities.html

[16] Harris, Susan. J. Nutr. 2006 Apr;136(4):1126-9. doi: 10.1093/jn/136.4.1126.

[17] Grant, W, et al. Evidence that Vitamin D Supplementation Could Reduce Risk of Influenza and COVID-19 Infections and Deaths. Nutrients. 12;988;April, 2, 2020. doi: 10.3390/nu12040988

[18] Grant, W. et al. IBID. 2020.

[19] Herr, C.; Shaykhiev, R.; Bals, R. The role of cathelicidin and defensins in pulmonary inflammatory diseases. Expert Opin. Biol. Ther. 2007, 7, 1449–1461

[20] Rondanelli, M, et al. Self-Care for Common Colds: The Pivotal Role of Vitamin D, Vitamin C, Zinc, and *Echinacea* in Three Main Immune Interactive Clusters (Physical Barriers, Innate and Adaptive Immunity) Involved during an Episode of Common Colds—Practical Advice on Dosages and on the Time to Take These Nutrients/Botanicals in order to Prevent or Treat Common Colds. Evidence-Based Complementary and Alternative Medicine : 2018; Article ID 5813095; https://doi.org/10.1155/2018/5813095

[21] Merzon, E, et al. Low plasma 25(OH) vitamin D level is associated with increased risk of COVID-19 infection: an Israeli population-based study. The FEBS Journal. July 23, 2020. https://doi.org/10.1111/febs.15495

[22] Accessed 7.29.20 from: https://www.medscape.com/viewarticle/934835?src=mkm_covid_update_200729_mscpedit_&uac=83217PG&impID=2482149&faf=1

[23] Novel, C.P.E.R.E. The epidemiological characteristics of an outbreak of 2019 novel coronavirus diseases (COVID-19) in China. Zhonghua Liu Xing Bing Xue Za Zhi 2020, 41, 145–151

[24] Vasarhelyi, B.; Satori, A.; Olajos, F.; Szabo, A.; Beko, G. Low vitamin D levels among patients at Semmelweis University: Retrospective analysis during a one-year period. Orv. Hetil. 2011, 152, 1272–1277

[25] Sharifi, A.; Vahedi, H.; Nedjat, S.; Rafiei, H.; Hosseinzadeh-Attar, M.J. Effect of single-dose injection of vitaminDonimmunecytokinesinulcerativecolitispatients: Arandomizedplacebo-controlledtrial. APMIS 2019, 127, 681–687.

[26] Gombart, A.F.; Pierre, A.; Maggini, S. A Review of Micronutrients and the Immune System-Working in Harmony to Reduce the Risk of Infection. Nutrients 2020, 12, 236

[27] Lemire, J.M.; Adams, J.S.; Kermani-Arab, V.; Bakke, A.C.; Sakai, R.; Jordan, S.C. 1,25-Dihydroxyvitamin D3 suppresses human T helper/inducer lymphocyte activity in vitro. J. Immunol. 1985, 134, 3032–3035

[28] Jeffery,L.E.;Burke,F.;Mura,M.;Zheng,Y.;Qureshi,O.S.;Hewison,M.;Walker,L.S.;Lammas,D.A.;Raza,K.; Sansom, D.M. 1,25-Dihydroxyvitamin D3 and IL-2 combine to inhibit T cell production of inflammatory cytokines and promote development of regulatory T cells expressing CTLA-4 and FoxP3. J. Immunol. 2009, 183, 5458–5467.

[29] Lei, G.S.; Zhang, C.; Cheng, B.H.; Lee, C.H. Mechanisms of Action of Vitamin D as Supplemental Therapy for Pneumocystis Pneumonia. Antimicrob. Agents Chemother. 2017, 61

[30] Brownstein, D, et al. A novel approach to treating COVID-19 Using nutritional and oxidative therapies. Science, Public Health Policy and The Law. Vol. 2:4-22. July 2020.

[31] Alipio, Mark, Vitamin D Supplementation Could Possibly Improve Clinical Outcomes of Patients Infected with Coronavirus-2019 (COVID-19) (April 9, 2020). Available at SSRN: https://ssrn.com/abstract=3571484 or http://dx.doi.org/10.2139/ssrn.3571484

[32] Kast, J.I., McFarlane, A.J., Głobińska, A., Sokolowska, M., Wawrzyniak, P., Sanak, M., Schwarze, J., Akdis, C.A. and Wanke, K. (2017), Respiratory syncytial virus infection influences tight junction integrity. Clin Exp Immunol, 190: 351-359. doi:10.1111/cei.13042

[33] Schwalfenberg GK. A review of the critical role of vitamin D in the functioning of the immune system and the clinical implications of vitamin D deficiency. *Mol Nutr Food Res*. 2011;55(1):96-108. doi:10.1002/mnfr.201000174

Chapter 6

Iodine

Iodine and Viruses

Carol is a 54-year-old advertising executive who became ill with a cough and shortness of breath. She said, "The symptoms became worse over a few days and then the fevers came. One minute I was a normal temperature, then I was at 102 degrees (Fahrenheit). This went on for a few days before I decided to call you. I told you what was going on and you asked me what I was taking. I said I was taking Tylenol® for the fever, and that was about it."

I had not seen Carol for over a year before her phone call. Carol told me she had not been taking any supplements for a few months because she had run out. I stated, "Well, you should be on our antiviral protocol of vitamins A, C, D, and iodine. It really helps out the immune system for patients sufferring with viral or bacterial infections." Carol told me that she still had iodine but not the others. I asked Carol to take 50 mg of Lugol's iodine daily for four days and that she should begin taking vitamins A, C, and D as per my protocol. I also stated, "Please don't use acetaminophen (Tylenol®) as it interferes with glutathione production and this can make any illness worse."

Carol immediately began taking iodine since she had it at home. The other supplements did not come for a few days. When I spoke to her several days later, Carol said, "The iodine was really great. A few hours after I started taking it, my mucus thinned out and I could cough up phlegm better. I felt better, too. The next day, after the second dose, I knew I was on the way to getting over this. I received the other supplements later in the third day and I took those for four days. But I was already better from the iodine. I will not forget to take iodine ever again."

Iodine is needed by the white blood cells to fight infections. Iodine has strong mucolytic properties. There is no bacteria or virus that has been shown to be resistant to iodine. Iodine deficiency is all-too-common across the country. Our body does not store iodine, so if you do not have enough in your diet or you stop supplementing with it, you will become deficient within 24–72 hours. My experience has been clear: I have yet to find a single nutrient that has provided as many positive effects on the body as iodine does.

Introduction

I have been researching, writing, and lecturing about iodine for over 20 years. I can state, with confidence, that it is the single most important nutrient that I have utilized in my practice. In my experience, iodine provides more bang for the buck than any other nutrient on the market.

For over 100 years, iodine has been known as the element that is necessary for thyroid hormone production. However, it is rare to see any mention of iodine's other effects in the body. Iodine is found in each of the trillions of cells in the body. Without adequate iodine levels, life itself is not possible.

Iodine is Needed to Produce Every Hormone

Iodine is not only necessary to produce thyroid hormones; it is also responsible for the production of all the other hormones in the body. Adequate iodine levels are necessary for proper immune system function. Iodine contains potent antibacterial, antiparasitic, antiviral, and anticancer properties. Iodine is also effective for treating fibrocystic breasts and ovarian cysts. Table 1 (next page) lists some of the many benefits of iodine and some of the conditions that benefit from adequate iodine supplementation.

Therapeutic Actions of Iodine

Approximately 1.5 billion people, about one-third of the earth's population, live in an area of iodine deficiency as defined by the World Health Organization. Iodine deficiency disorder can result in intellectual disability, goiter, increased child and infant mortality, infertility, and socioeconomic decline.[1] Iodine deficiency disorder is the most common preventable form of intellectual disability known.

Table 1: Therapeutic Actions of Iodine and Conditions Iodine Can Treat

Therapeutic Actions	Conditions Treated with Iodine
Antibacterial	ADD/ADHD
Anticancer	Atherosclerosis
Antiparasitic	Breast Diseases
Antiviral	Dupuytren's Contracture
Elevates pH	Excess Mucus Production
Mucolytic Agent	Fatigue
	Fibrocystic Breasts
	Goiter
	Hemorrhoids
	Headaches and Migraine Headaches
	Hypertension
	Infections
	Keloids
	Liver Diseases
	Nephrotic Syndrome
	Ovarian Disease
	Pancreatic Disorders
	Parotid Duct Stones
	Peyronie's
	Prostate Disorders
	Sebaceous Cysts
	Skin lesions
	Thyroid Disorders
	Vaginal Infections

Iodine Deficiency: How Common Is It?

In the United States, iodine deficiency is far too common. For over 40 years, US iodine levels have fallen in the National Health and Nutrition Examination Survey (NHANES).[2]

Nearly 60% of women of childbearing age are deficient in iodine.[3] In fact, the latest mean urinary iodine concentration among pregnant US women is 134 ug/L, which signifies deficiency.[4]

Iodine is a relatively rare element, ranking 62nd in abundance of the elements of the earth. It is estimated to be about 0.3-0.5 parts per million. This puts it in the bottom third of the elements in terms of abundance.[5]

Iodine is primarily found in seawater in small quantities and in solid rocks (usually near the ocean) that form when seawater evaporates. Iodine can also be found in sea organisms, such as seaweed. In fact, seaweed is one of the most abundant sources of iodine because seaweed has the ability to concentrate a large amount of iodine from ocean water.

If soil has adequate iodine levels, the crops grown on that soil will contain adequate iodine levels. Conversely, deficient iodine levels will be found in crops grown on iodine-deficient soil, with potential impacts on human health.

Different Forms of Iodine

Naturally occurring iodine is non-radioactive. Radioactive iodine has been manufactured for medical and industrial uses. In medicine, radioactive iodine has been used to diagnose and treat certain illnesses, particularly illnesses of the thyroid gland. However, only naturally occurring, non-radioactive iodine is considered a nutrient or used as a dietary supplement.

Commercially available iodine primarily comes from several sources: Chilean saltpeter, seaweed, and brine water in oil wells. The action of the waves from the ocean can make iodine gas. Once airborne, iodine can combine with water or air and enter the soil. Iodine can enter our food system in a variety of ways. First, plants can take up iodine from the soil. Second, airborne iodine can land on fresh water supplies or land on the ground for plant uptake. Iodine also finds its way into the human diet through seafood, sea vegetables, and in commercially prepared iodized salt.

Radioactive iodine can enter the air from reactions in nuclear power plants or explosions of nuclear materials. Radioactive iodine has been associated with certain types of cancer, including thyroid cancer and certain blood cancers. Children are more susceptible to radioactive iodine since they have smaller thyroid glands, and they will receive a proportionately larger radioactive dose than an adult when they are exposed to radioactive iodine. Radioactive iodine damage can be prevented by the ingestion of non-radioactive, inorganic iodine.

My book, *Iodine: Why You Need It, Why You Can't Live Without It*, provides more information about iodine's effects in the body. In this book, I will focus on how iodine affects the immune system and particularly how maintaining adequate iodine levels can provide protection against infectious organisms.

Iodine and Iodide

Different tissues in the body preferentially utilize either the oxidized or reduced forms of iodine. Some of this is complex, but I will do my best to help you understand this important topic as it relates to the antiviral, antibacterial, and anti-parasitic effects of iodine.

Iodine refers to the oxidized form of iodide. Iodide refers to the reduced form of iodine. The terms oxidation and reduction are chemical terms that relate to the number of electrons in the outer shell of an element. When iodine has a full complement of electrons in the outer shell, it is referred to as iodide—the reduced form. When the same molecule is lacking an electron, in other words, when there is an unpaired electron in the outer shell, it is then termed iodine, which is the oxidized form of iodide.

Iodine and iodide have quite different effects in the body. Iodide binds to thyroid tissue and is utilized to manufacture thyroid hormone. Iodine, the oxidized form that is lacking an electron in its outer shell, has direct anti-pathogenic organism effects, including antiviral capabilities.

Iodine as an Antiviral Agent

It has been known for over 70 years that iodine not only has potent antiviral abilities but also functions as a broad range antiseptic agent as well. In our modern world, iodine is still used prior to surgery to sterilize the skin.

The 1918 Influenza Pandemic killed an estimated 30 million people worldwide. When the H1N1 influenza virus was established as the pathogen, a search was undertaken to find out how to prevent this virus, as well as future viruses, from causing the same type of deadly pandemic from happening again. Scientists searched for substances that would destroy the virus. At that time, iodine was identified as one of the most effective antiviral agents.

In 1945, three Australian researchers, F.M. Burnett, H.F. Holden and J.D. Stone studied the effects of iodine, especially iodine mists, on influenza viruses.[6] Mice were studied as mice were shown to be readily infected by exposure for a short period to a mist of influenza virus droplets. The researchers painted iodine on the snouts of mice and found it protected the mice from infection when the mice were exposed to live influenza virus from a mist. Iodine was found to be a potent inactivating agent to the influenza virus. The scientists reported, "Perhaps the most striking of the early experiments was the demonstration that mice could be protected completely merely by painting a little tincture of iodine on their snouts several minutes before they were...exposed to a concentration of mist capable of producing heavy infection or death {from influenza virus} in control mice."[7]

Iodine, the Immune System, and Antisepsis

Iodine is also an essential agent for our immune system. In fact, our immune system cannot function optimally without iodine. Iodine supplementation has been shown to increase IgG (immunoglobulin G) synthesis in human lymphocytes.[8] IgG is utilized by the immune system to provide long-term and often lifelong immunity to various infectious organisms. As described in Chapter 2, the white blood cells are part of the innate immune system and are known as first-responders when an infectious agent has been identified in the body. The white blood cells remove pathogens by engulfing and destroying them. This is known as phagocytosis. Iodine deficiency is associated with decreased phagocytic activity of blood neutrophils.[9] Iodine has been shown to increase the ability of white blood cells to kill infectious organisms.[10]

Iodine is also used as an antiseptic throughout the US because it has antiviral and antibacterial properties. I have utilized iodine as an effective antiviral and antiseptic agent for over two decades.

To reduce transmission of viruses, antisepsis of human and non-human surfaces must be identified. Researchers reported an *in vitro* study where SARS-CoV-2, the cause of the COVID-19 pandemic, was exposed to iodine (povidone-iodine) at 1-5% concentrations as a nasal antiseptic formulation and an oral rinse. The iodine solutions effectively inactivated SARS-CoV-2 after exposure times of 60 seconds.[11] In vitro studies of 0.23% povidone-iodine (PVP-I) mouthwash (1:30 dilution) was shown to inactivate both SARS-CoV-2 and MERS-CoV (Middle East Respiratory Syndrome) following a 15-second exposure.[12]

Japan has one of the lowest rates of COVID-19 illness in the world, including the crowded city of Tokyo. Furthermore, Japan has not gone on a total lockdown. The Japanese are known to have a much higher iodine intake through their diet compared to other countries. It is estimated that the mainland Japanese ingest over 100x the RDA as compared to US citizens.[13] Perhaps Tokyo and Japan have had fewer serious COVID-19 illnesses because of their iodine intake.

Final Thoughts

In my COVID-19 study,[14] iodine was used both as a

nebulized solution and orally. COVID-19 patients were advised to take 25 mg per day of a combination of iodine and iodide in the form of Lugol's 5% solution (4 drops) or tableted Lugol's solution. Nebulized iodine in a dilute solution of hydrogen peroxide was also utilized. When nebulizing iodine, I have my patients use one drop of 5% Lugol's solution in 3cc of a dilute hydrogen peroxide mixture. More about this can be found in my published paper (referenced above) and in the Appendix, and more about nebulizing can be found in Chapter 9.

I have over 20 years of clinical experience using iodine as both an oral supplement and as a nebulized solution. In my opinion, properly prescribed iodine should be part of any antiviral (as well as antibacterial, anti-parasitic and antifungal) regimen. In fact, maintaining optimal iodine levels should be part of any health regimen. The results I have seen have been truly remarkable. I was not surprised in the least when iodine along with vitamins A, C, D as well as ozone and hydrogen peroxide quickly helped my COVID-19 patients recover.

Iodine is a relatively safe supplement to take. There are few side effects when it is used appropriately. As with any natural therapy, it is best to work with a holistic doctor who is iodine-literate. More information about iodine can be found in my book, *Iodine: Why You Need It, Why You Can't Live Without It, 5ᵗʰ Edition.*

[1] Manner, M.G., et al. Salt Iodization for the Elimination of Iodine Deficiency. International Council for the Control of Iodine Deficiency Disorders. 1995

[2] Cdc.gov. 2020. *Second National Report On Biochemical Indicators Of Diet And Nutrition In The U.S. Population.* [online] Available at: <http://www.cdc.gov/nutritionreport/pdf/Nutrition_Book_complete508_final.pdf#zoom=100> [Accessed 7 June 2020].

[3] Caldwell, K., Makhmudov, A., Ely, E., Jones, R. and Wang, R., 2011. Iodine Status of the U.S. Population, National Health and Nutrition Examination Survey, 2005–2006 and 2007–2008. *Thyroid*, 21(4), pp.419-427.

[4] Kathleen L. Caldwell, Yi Pan, Mary E. Mortensen, Amir Makhmudov, Lori Merrill, and John Moye.Thyroid.Aug 2013.927-937.http://doi.org/10.1089/thy.2013.0012

[5] Modern Nutrition in Health and Disease, 9th Edition. Williams and Wilkins, 1999.

[6] Burnet, FM, Holden, HF, and Stone, JD. Action of iodine vapour on influenza virus in droplet suspension. *Aust J Sci.* 1945;7:125.

[7] Burnet, FM, Holden, HF, and Stone. IBID. 1945.

[8] Weetman AP, McGregor AM, Campbell H, Lazarus JH, Ibbertson HK, Hall R. Iodide enhances IgG synthesis by human peripheral blood lymphocytes in vitro. *Acta Endocrinol (Copenh).* 1983;103(2):210-215. doi:10.1530/acta.0.1030210

[9] Zel'tser ME. Vliianie khronicheskogo defitsita ĭoda v ratsione na razvitie infektsionnogo protsessa [Effect of a chronic iodine deficit in the ration on the development of the infectious process]. *Zh Mikrobiol Epidemiol Immunobiol.* 1975;0(9):116-119.

[10] Venturi S, Venturi M. Iodine, thymus, and immunity. *Nutrition.* 2009;25(9):977-979. doi:10.1016/j.nut.2009.06.002

[11] Pelletier, J., Tessema, B., Westover, J., Frank, S., Brown, S. and Capriotti, J., 2020. In Vitro Efficacy of Povidone-Iodine Nasal And Oral Antiseptic Preparations Against Severe Acute Respiratory Syndrome-Coronavirus 2 (SARS-CoV-2).

[12] Eggers M, Koburger-Janssen T, Eickmann M, Zorn J. In Vitro Bactericidal and Virucidal Efficacy of Povidone-Iodine Gargle/Mouthwash Against Respiratory and Oral Tract Pathogens. *Infect Dis Ther.* 2018;7(2):249-259. doi:10.1007/s40121-018-0200-7

[13] Abraham, G., Flechas, J. and Hakala, J., n.d. *Orthoiodosupplementation: Iodine Sufficiency Of The Whole Human Body.* [online] Optimox.com. Available at: <https://www.optimox.com/iodine-study-2>

[14] Brownstein, D., et al. A Novel Approach to Treating COVID-19 with Nutritional and Oxidative Therapies. Science, Public Health Policy, and The Law Volume 2:4-22 July, 2020 Clinical and Translational Research.

Chapter 7

Hydrogen Peroxide

Hydrogen Peroxide

Jack is a 71-year-old retired carpenter. He became ill at the beginning of the COVID-19 crises in the Detroit metropolitan area in March 2020. Jack was following my blog posts about COVID-19 and was concerned when he started coughing and developed a low-grade fever. "I felt terrible," Jack said. "I have had the flu before, and this started off the same way. I had body aches and pains, a headache and a fever, with my temperature going from 100 to 103 degrees."

Jack began taking the oral vitamins A, C, D, and iodine in the large doses I was writing about. However, he kept feeling worse. After seven days of worsening symptoms and now having a productive cough, Jack went to the emergency room. He was diagnosed with bilateral pneumonia and placed on IV antibiotics and oxygen. After four days of therapy, Jack's PCR test for SARS-CoV-2 came back positive. At this point his doctors stopped the IV antibiotics and treated him solely with oxygen.

"I was not feeling better and the doctors kept saying that there was nothing more they could do for me," he said. For three days, Jack sat in his hospital room in isolation, only receiving oxygen. He said, *"At this point, I told them to send me home as I was not getting better or worse. I felt like if I stayed there, something bad was going to happen to me."*

Jack was discharged home and immediately called me. I have treated Jack for over 20 years and know him well. I would not have recognized his voice if I did not know it was him on the line. Jack sounded very weak and could barely speak. He told me in a tearful voice, *"I am going to die."*

I told Jack to forget that thought. I stated, *"My partners and I have treated many patients with similar symptoms. They have gotten better, and I don't see why you can't, too. Why don't you come to our parking lot for intravenous doses of hydrogen peroxide and vitamin C as well as intramuscular shots of ozone."*

Jack declined. *"I am too weak to travel,"* he stated.

I suggested that he go back to the emergency room, but he refused, saying he would rather die at home. At this point, I asked to speak to his wife. I suggested that she come to our office to pick up a nebulizer and hydrogen peroxide nebulizing solution. I instructed her to have Jack nebulize 3cc of dilute hydrogen peroxide along with a drop of 5% Lugol's iodine every hour until he felt better, *then back off gradually. I said we would talk at the end of the day. Jack called me after the second nebulizer treatment. He said, "I can't believe it. After the first nebulized treatment the pain and tightness in my chest began to ease a little bit. This was the first time I had felt better in over a week. After the second dose, one hour later, it was a miracle. My lungs opened and I could breathe again. I do not know how to thank you. You saved my life," Jack stated this through tears.*

I shed some tears too at that moment. Jack is a strong man. I had never heard him talk like this. I told Jack to continue nebulizing and reduce the frequency as he felt better. It took Jack three days to feel close to normal.

Jack's story is not unique. As I stated in the first chapter, this holistic protocol for treating viral and other pathogenic organisms has been used for over 25 years. I have been recommending nebulized peroxide for nearly this entire time period. I have seen wonderful results for those suffering from many different lung issues, including chronic obstructive pulmonary disease (COPD), fibrosis of the lungs, bronchitis, and pneumonia.

Introduction

Hydrogen peroxide can be identified by its chemical structure: H_2O_2. Figure 1 (next page) shows a structural diagram of hydrogen peroxide.

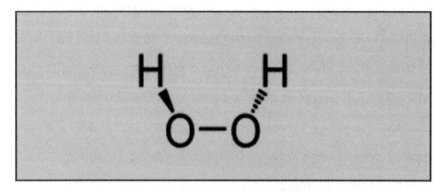

Figure 1: Structure of Hydrogen Peroxide

As you can see from the chemical structure, each molecule of hydrogen peroxide contains two atoms of hydrogen and two atoms of oxygen. It is basically a water molecule, (H_2O) with one additional oxygen atom (H_2O_2). Concentrated hydrogen peroxide is a colorless liquid that can explode if heated. It is a highly volatile substance that is used as a propellant in rocket fuel, and also finds applications in manufacturing processes. Hydrogen peroxide for home use is diluted with water and safe to handle. Tiny quantities of hydrogen peroxide are found in rainwater as well as snow. It is thought to occur naturally as a product of ozone, when it descends from the atmosphere and encounters water vapor.[1] [2]

Hydrogen peroxide was first synthesized in the lab by the French scientist Louis Jacques Thenard in 1818. He was a French chemist who studied pharmacy in Paris and later became a professor of chemistry. Thenard was working with barium peroxide when he noticed, by accident, that hydrogen peroxide was created as a byproduct when barium peroxide was added to water. He called hydrogen peroxide *eau oxygene*, or "oxygen water". Thenard's method of producing hydrogen peroxide remained the most common production method until the mid-twentieth century.

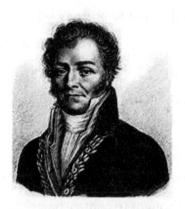

Louis Jacques Thenard
(1777-1857)

Hydrogen Peroxide in the Human Body

Hydrogen peroxide is continually produced in the human body. In fact, every cell in the body is exposed to some level of hydrogen peroxide.[3] The mitochondria, the energy producing organelles of the body, generate substantial amounts of hydrogen peroxide.[4]

Oral bacteria produce hydrogen peroxide to control the growth of certain bacterial strains.[5] [6] It is also produced in the ocular tissues.

Hydrogen peroxide is also present in the exhaled air of healthy humans as well as those with lung diseases.[7] Hydrogen peroxide is produced in the lungs.[8] Although it is uncertain where the lungs produce hydrogen peroxide, it is thought that white blood cells (polymorphonuclear cells or PMNs—part of the body's innate defense cells) in the lungs may be producing it in order to control bacterial growth. This may explain why those with inflammatory lung diseases and cigarette smokers have greater amounts of exhaled hydrogen peroxide compared to normal subjects.[9]

Hydrogen peroxide is also found in large quantities in human urine and is thought to control bacterial growth in the urine. In addition, researchers also believe that hydrogen peroxide is continually produced in the bloodstream.

One of the main effects of hydrogen peroxide production in the human body is to signal an alarm when a tissue has been injured. As a result of locally increased production of hydrogen peroxide, the body's defense cells—white blood cells—are signaled to come to the aid.

Production of Hydrogen Peroxide Stimulates Many Biochemical Processes

Hydrogen peroxide acts as a "second messenger" in many

biological processes. This includes stimulating both anti-inflammatory and pro-inflammatory molecules, including nuclear factor kB.

Hydrogen peroxide also stimulates fibroblast proliferation and new blood vessel growth,[10] [11] and can activate lymphocytes, the white blood cells designed to fight viral and other infections.[12] It is important to note that lymphocytes are often depleted in viral infections. COVID-19 is characterized by lymphocyte depletion. It is further known to stimulate the production of nitric oxide, which has powerful effects on the vascular system of the body.[13]

Hydrogen Peroxide and Infections

Hydrogen peroxide has been used for generations as an antiviral and antibacterial agent. In American households, it is commonplace to have hydrogen peroxide available for use after an injury that results in a laceration of the skin. In this situation, hydrogen peroxide is poured into the wound to sterilize it and help prevent infection.

In wounds, hydrogen peroxide works by moistening and loosening debris in a wound. It can also directly disable a viral or bacterial pathogen but does not work against all pathogenic strains.

As I explained in my COVID-19 paper, when H_2O_2 is produced extracellularly or added to a cell culture system, a gradient of H_2O_2 is quickly established across the plasma membrane.[14] Researchers reported that the gradient is the result of H_2O_2-scavanging enzymes, including catalase and GSH-peroxidase, which maintain a steady-state intracellular H_2O_2 concentration being 10x less than the extracellular concentration.[15] As Bocci states, "This result is important because the intravenous (IV) infusion of a low and calculated concentration of H_2O_2 results in a marked dilution in the plasma pool with partial inactivation and in intracellular levels able to exert biological effects on blood and endothelial cells without aggravating the concomitant oxidative stress."[16] COVID-19 is known to cause oxidative stress, which may be the cause of multi-organ failure and hypoxemia.[17] [18] [19] H_2O_2 is known to activate glycolysis, ATP and 2,3-DPG in red blood cells which can lead to improved oxygen delivery to ischemic (blood deficient) tissues.[20] [21] H_2O_2 has also been shown to increase the production of nitric oxide (NO), which can aid in vasodilation and tissue oxygenation.[22] [23]

Coronaviruses have been shown to be sensitive to oxidizing disinfectants such as a 0.5% hydrogen peroxide solution used as a surface disinfectant.[24] It is well accepted that the response of the immune system to infection involves the production of pro-oxidants, which are known to disinfect pathogens.[25]

Nebulized and Intravenous Hydrogen Peroxide

In my practice, I utilize hydrogen peroxide therapy via both nebulizing (inhaled) and intravenous routes. This section will review the physiology of how hydrogen peroxide works. The specifics of the concentration and 'how to do it' will be covered in the nebulizing and intravenous therapy chapters.

As previously mentioned, the lungs continually produce hydrogen peroxide. Nebulized hydrogen peroxide has been shown to have antiviral activities.[26] Hydrogen peroxide can activate certain white blood cells—lymphocytes—which are known to be depleted in COVID-19 and in other infections.[27]

My partners and I have successfully used nebulized peroxide for treating lung diseases for over 20 years. In fact, the use of nebulized peroxide is one of the safest and most effective regimens for lung problems that I have seen. The lung conditions we have treated with nebulized (and intravenous) peroxide include:

- Bronchitis
- Chronic Obstructive Pulmonary Disease
- Pneumonia
- Pulmonary fibrosis
- Upper respiratory infections

- Viral infections

I have also utilized intravenous dosing of hydrogen peroxide for the above bulleted conditions. Hydrogen peroxide and ozone have similar physiological effects in the body.

Early Medical Uses of Hydrogen Peroxide

To understand how effective hydrogen peroxide is in treating infectious illnesses, I think it is important to go back and look at the pioneers of this therapy.

The medical uses of hydrogen peroxide were first reported by Dr. T.H. Oliver and colleagues in 1920. Dr. Oliver was a British physician stationed in India. In 1919, he reported a severe epidemic of influenza and fatal broncho-pneumonia, which was afflicting Indian troops.[28] His report states, "It was unfortunately impossible to give statistics of the mortality of the epidemic, but its extent may be gauged from the fact that in one large Indian hospital in which influenza cases were segregated in special huts the death-rate was over 80% in the pneumonia cases with toxic symptoms."

Dr. Oliver was frustrated with the treatments available to him. He wrote, "So useless were the usual remedies tried in [these patients] that we felt justified in giving a trial to any method which held out a prospect of success. It had been observed by one of us (Dr. Oliver) some years previously that [a solution] of hydrogen peroxide had, in the presence of a catalyst (copper) a remarkable oxidizing power…" [29] [30] Furthermore, Dr. Oliver wrote, "Further investigation, as yet unpublished, showed that many other substances were similarly oxidized {sic} by this solution, the power of which appeared to depend primarily on the formation of nascent oxygen."

Dr. Oliver could have been describing the effects of using ozone since hydrogen peroxide and ozone share many of the same mechanisms of action, including increasing the oxygenation of the tissues of the body.

Dr. Oliver continued by stating, "We thought that use might be made of this reaction if the H_2O_2 were given intravenously, in this instance employing the well-known catalytic powers of haemoblogin [sic] as a substitute for the copper, and we hoped thereby, not only to supply oxygen to the tissues with greater rapidity than by the ordinary methods, but also to render the circulating toxins inert by oxidation."

First Use of Intravenous Hydrogen Peroxide to Treat Pneumonia

Dr. Oliver went on to describe the effect of intravenous hydrogen peroxide on his Indian patients. The first patient was suffering from pneumonia and was "intensely toxic". (I assume Dr. Oliver meant the patient was very ill with sepsis or bacteria in the bloodstream). The patient was selected as the worst case in the ward and had been delirious for two days prior. Dr. Oliver administered a dilute solution of hydrogen peroxide into the patient for fifteen minutes. Over the course of ten days, the soldier gradually improved. Dr. Oliver wrote, "The change in the mental condition was remarkable, the patient, who previously had had to be tied in bed owing to delirium, was within six hours of the injection sitting up and asking for food; he slept well the next night and from that time improved in every way, eventually being invalided to India as a walking case three weeks later."

Dr. Oliver was encouraged by his first patient's response to intravenous hydrogen peroxide. He then tried the same hydrogen peroxide infusion on 24 other soldiers who suffered with pneumonia. Dr. Oliver's team only selected the sickest patients. Of the 25 subjects treated, 13 recovered and 12 died, a mortality rate of 48%. This rate is compared to the 80% death rate from the usual care offered at that time.

The conclusion of the article stated, "From our experience, we conclude:

1.   Hydrogen peroxide can be given intravenously without gas embolism being produced.
2.   The anoxaemia [sic]–low oxygen symptoms–is often markedly benefited.

3. The toxaemia [sic]–spread of bacterial products in the blood stream–appears to be overcome in many cases.

4. The mortality (48%) [with hydrogen peroxide therapy] compares very favorably with the 80% mortality in similar cases not so treated, and more so when it is remembered that we only treated the most severe and apparently hopeless."

You would think that Dr. Oliver's research results with using hydrogen peroxide would have sparked widespread interest in other doctors. However, when antibiotics were introduced and promoted in the conventional medical world, the interest in hydrogen peroxide therapy plummeted, especially since hydrogen peroxide was not patentable. It is astounding to me that to this day, hydrogen peroxide therapy is virtually unknown in conventional medicine.

The Ozone–Hydrogen Peroxide Connection

Dr. Velio Bocci, et. al, found that the ozonation of human plasma triggers a reaction leading to the release of hydrogen peroxide.[31] [32] Ozonated serum added to human cell cultures further induces a significant and steady increase in nitric oxide (NO).[33] [34] Nitric oxide is an important signaling molecule that has many physiological properties such as vasodilation (dilating the blood vessels to increase blood flow). When hydrogen peroxide is introduced along with ozone therapy, there is a rapid increase in NO formation.[35]

Dr. Bocci has stated, "Physiological concentrations of [hydrogen peroxide] can trigger several biochemical pathways without deleterious effects because the normal cell has an efficacious antioxidant capacity that rapidly reduces {hydrogen peroxide} to water."[36] Furthermore, Dr. Bocci claims that hydrogen peroxide is an "early and effective ozone messenger."

The physiological and biochemical effects of hydrogen peroxide in the body are thus very similar to those of ozone. Because of this, hydrogen peroxide and ozone therapies share similar positive outcomes. These include:

- Activating the immune system to fight infection
- Improving oxygen delivery to tissues
- Stimulating ATP production and NO production
- Up-regulating antioxidant enzymes

Hydrogen Peroxide: A Potent Antibacterial Substance

It is well known that hydrogen peroxide has an antibacterial effect.[37] White blood cells, particularly the polymorphonuclear leukocytes (PMNs), are responsible for mediating the fight against pathogenic bacteria. PMNs can generate hydrogen peroxide and other substances to kill foreign invaders.

Researchers have found that hydrogen peroxide can significantly reduce the number of bacteria in culture.[38] It is thought that the widespread production of hydrogen peroxide in the human body is done, in part, to provide balance between native bacteria and pathogenic bacteria.

The Connection Between Vitamin C and Hydrogen Peroxide

It is well known that vitamin C has many health benefits in the human body. In fact, vitamin C is an essential nutrient for humans since the human body cannot manufacture it. If we do not take in enough vitamin C, associated illnesses like scurvy, heart disease and even death can occur.

Many holistically oriented health care providers utilize oral and intravenous doses of vitamin C in their practice. I have successfully used intravenous vitamin C for over 20 years.

One of vitamin C's potent effects, or perhaps its most potent effect, is to stimulate the production of hydrogen peroxide—just as ozone does. Intravenous vitamin C has been shown to cause a marked increase in hydrogen peroxide production.[39] In fact, the positive effects that intravenous vitamin C produce may, in fact, be mostly related to the increased production of hydrogen peroxide and the resultant increased oxygenation of the body's tissues. Therefore, simultaneously giving ill patients hydrogen peroxide and vitamin C along with ozone could provide a synergistic effect. That is exactly what I have seen in my career. That is why I chose to use a combination of intravenous vitamin C and hydrogen peroxide along with intramuscular ozone shots to my patients ill with a viral pathogen.

Adverse Effects of Hydrogen Peroxide Therapy

My experience, after giving thousands of hydrogen peroxide IVs as well as nebulized H_2O_2 for inhalation, is that there are very few adverse effects when hydrogen peroxide is properly administered. In fact, hydrogen peroxide therapy is one of the safest treatments I have witnessed. The most common adverse event reported in the literature is irritation and sclerosis (hardening) as well as disappearing of the vein it is injected into. However, I can state that, when properly administered, vein problems from intravenous hydrogen peroxide therapy are very rare. I cannot recall one case where a patient's vein disappeared due to intravenous use of hydrogen peroxide. Perhaps my practice partners and I see a lowered rate of side effects because we use low-dose hydrogen peroxide for our infusions and nebulizer treatments. This is further discussed in Chapter 9.

Final Thoughts

Hydrogen peroxide therapy, when done correctly, is very safe. I have found it to be one of the most effective anti-pathogenic therapies I have used in my practice. In fact, I consider it my 'go to' therapy when a patient is acutely ill with a pathogenic organism, whether it be viral, bacterial, parasitic or fungal. When I personally find myself in the first stages of an illness, the first therapy I reach for is hydrogen peroxide.

As part of an antiviral regimen, I consider hydrogen peroxide therapy invaluable. In the cases of COVID-19 that I treated, I consistently heard from my patients that they felt nebulizing hydrogen peroxide made a dramatic improvement in their condition. I was not surprised, as I have been observing this in my practice for over 20 years. More about nebulizing hydrogen peroxide can be found in Chapter 9.

[1] Ann Chim. 2003 Apr;93(4):477-88

[2] Atmospheric Environment. Vol. 30, No. 6. 967:1996

[3] FEBS Letters
Volume 486, Issue 1, 1 December 2000, Pages 10–13

[4] Physiological Reviews. Vol. 59. 3:1979:527

[5] Arch. Oral Biol., 40 (1995), pp. 753–763

[6] J. Oral. Pathol., 16 (1987), pp. 412–416

[7] Journal of Biological Chemistry
Volume 258, Issue 6, 1983, Pages 3628-3631

[8] Rysz J, Stolarek RA, Luczynski R, and et al. Increased hydrogen peroxide concentration in the exhaled breath condensate of stable COPD patients after nebulized N-acetylcysteine . Pulm Pharmacol Ther., 20(3):281-289, 2007.

[9] Chest, 96 (1989), pp. 606–612

[10] Life Sci 64: 249-258, 1999

[11] Free Radic. Biol. Med 25: 891-897, 1998

[12] Nat.Immunol 3: 1129-1134, 2002

[13] Rivista Italiana di Ossigeno-Ozonoterapia 4: 30-39, 2005

[14] Antunes, F. and Cadenas, E., 2000. Estimation of H2O2 gradients across biomembranes. *FEBS Letters*, 475(2), pp.121-126.

[15] James R. Stone & Tucker Collins (2002) The Role of Hydrogen Peroxide in Endothelial Proliferative Responses, Endothelium, 9:4, 231-238, DOI: 10.1080/10623320214733

[16] Bocci, V. & Aldinucci, Carlo & Bianchi, L.. (2005). The use of hydrogen peroxide as a medical drug. Rivista Italiana di Ossigeno-Ozonoterapia. 4. 30-39.

[17] Clinicaltrials.gov. 2020. *Correlation Between Oxidative Stress Status And COVID-19 Severity.* [online] Available at:
<https://clinicaltrials.gov/ct2/show/NCT04375137>

[18] Zhang C, Wu Z, Li J, Zhao H, Wang G. Cytokine release syndrome in severe COVID-19: interleukin-6 receptor antagonist tocilizumab may be the key to reduce mortality. *Int J Antimicrob Agents.* 2020;55(5):105954. doi:10.1016/j.ijantimicag.2020.105954

[19] Bermejo-Martin J, Almansa R, Menéndez R, Mendez R, Kelvin D, Torres A. Lymphopenic community acquired pneumonia as signature of severe COVID-19 infection. *Journal of Infection.* 2020;80(5):e23-e24. doi:10.1016/j.jinf.2020.02.029

[20] Bocci V. *Oxygen-Ozone Therapy.* Dordrecht: Springer; 2002:1440.

[21] Bocci V. *Ozone - A New Medical Drug.* 2nd ed. Dordrecht: Springer Netherlands; 2011:1-295.

[22] Valacchi G, Bocci V. Studies on the biological effects of ozone: 11. Release of factors from human endothelial cells. *Mediators Inflamm.* 2000;9(6):271-276. doi:10.1080/09629350020027573

[23] Thengchaisri N, Kuo L. Hydrogen peroxide induces endothelium-dependent and -independent coronary arteriolar dilation: role of cyclooxygenase and potassium channels. *American Journal of Physiology-Heart and Circulatory Physiology.* 2003;285(6):H2255-H2263. doi:10.1152/ajpheart.00487.2003

[24] Kampf G, Todt D, Pfaender S, Steinmann E. Persistence of coronaviruses on inanimate surfaces and their inactivation with biocidal agents. *Journal of Hospital Infection.* 2020;104(3):246-251. doi:10.1016/j.jhin.2020.01.022

[25] Open Journal of Molecular and Integrative Physiology
Vol.05 No.03(2015), Article ID:61563,12 pages
10.4236/ojmip.2015.53004

[26] Zonta W, Mauroy A, Farnir F, and Thiry E. Virucidal Efficacy of a Hydrogen Peroxide Nebulization Against Murine Norovirus and Feline Calicivirus, Two Surrogates of Human Norovirus . Food Environ Virol., 8(4):275-282, 2016.

[27] M Reth. Hydrogen peroxide as second messenger in lymphocyte activation . Nat Immunol 3, page 1129–1134, 2002

[28] The Lancet. Feb. 21, 1920. p. 432

[29] The Lancet. Feb 21, 1920. p. 432

[30] Medical Chronicle. July, 1914.

[31] Bocci V: Ozone.A new medical drug. Springer, Dordrecht, The Netherlands: 2004, 1-295

[32] Oxygen-ozone therapy. A critical evaluation. 1-440, Kluwer Academic Publishers, Dordrecht, The Netherlands, 2002.

[33] Mediators.Inflamm 9: 271-276, 2000

[34] Rivista Italiana di Ossigeno-Ozonoterapia 4: 30-39, 2005

[35] IBID. [35] Rivista Italiana di Ossigeno-Ozonoterapia 4: 30-39, 2005

[36] Rivista Italiana di Ossigeno-Ozonoterapia 4: 30-39, 2005

[37] Free Rad. Biology and Medicine. Vol. 19, 1:July, 1995:31

[38] Biochem. J. 254:685-92:1988

[39] Proceedings of the National Academy of Sciences of the USA. Vol. 104.221:8749. 2007

Chapter 8

Ozone

Ozone

Shelly is a 48-year-old homemaker. She became ill with a cough, fever (temperature 100-102 degrees Fahrenheit), sore throat, as well as body aches and pains. Since this was at the beginning of the COVID-19 pandemic that hit the Metro Detroit area, she called my office in a panic. "I am so scared. This all started last night and I don't know what to do. I called my internist and he told me to take Tylenol® and drink fluids. I know you have been writing about why not to take Tylenol® so I didn't take it. I feel like I am dying," she said.

I have known Shelly for many years. I remarked to her, "You sound sick, but you don't sound like you are dying. Why do you think you are dying?"

Shelly stated, "I am just so scared from what I see on T.V. People are dying from COVID-19."

I told Shelly that most people who died had co-morbidities, which she did not have. Furthermore, I said, "And, we have a good treatment plan that can help your immune system overcome a viral illness. Shelly was instructed to take the oral supplement regimen as described in this book—vitamins A, C, D, and iodine. I also asked her to begin nebulizing and to come in for intravenous infusions of vitamin C, hydrogen peroxide and intramuscular shots of ozone if she was not feeling better, or started feeling worse.

"I want to come in for everything," she said, "I just don't want to get sicker." I met Shelly in the parking lot at my office. Unfortunately for both of us—especially me—it was snowing outside at the time. I was wearing a face mask and full personal protection equipment. I remember having to shake the snow off my face mask, like a dog shakes his head, in order to put the IV in. Shelly was dehydrated, and the combination of her dehydration and the cold weather prevented me from giving her the IV therapies. Therefore, Shelly only received two intramuscular shots of ozone— at 18 gamma—in her buttocks.

I called Shelly at the end of the day and she was feeling much better. "It was a miracle," she said. "As I was driving home, I felt better. I could not believe it. The pressure on my head and the fever just went away, and I was able to eat again. Now, I know I am on the way to getting over this."

Shelly was tested later for COVID-19, which came back positive.

Shelly's story fit the pattern that became the norm for our COVID-19 patients: Most improved right away. Since Shelly did not receive the intravenous hydrogen peroxide or vitamin C, I attribute her quick recovery to the intramuscular shots of ozone. Over the years, I have seen many patients dramatically improve from the symptoms of a viral infection with the use of ozone.

Introduction

Ozone is a colorless gas with a pungent odor. It is a natural molecule made up of three atoms of oxygen. In contrast, the oxygen in the air we breathe is made up of two oxygen atoms. See Figure 1.

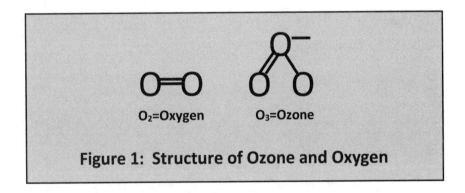

O_2=Oxygen O_3=Ozone

Figure 1: Structure of Ozone and Oxygen

The molecular weight of the oxygen molecule is 32; for ozone, with its extra oxygen atom, the molecular weight is 48.

Ozone has an overall negative charge—which means it is an oxidative molecule.

Ozone is also much more soluble in water than oxygen. 49.0 ml of ozone will dissolve in 100 ml of water, while the same amount of water will hold only 4.9 ml oxygen — a ten-fold difference in solubility.[1] The practical aspect of ozone's high solubility is that it makes this highly reactive substance easily absorbable in biological fluids—and thus the human body.

Ozone is produced by combining oxygen molecules. In the presence of an electric charge, O_2 (the oxygen molecule) is converted into O_3 (the ozone molecule) as shown below in Figure 2. Notice that the reaction shown in Figure 2 is reversible. This chemical equation shows that three molecules of oxygen, when exposed to an electrical spark, convert into two molecules of ozone. Likewise, ozone, once produced, can spontaneously revert back to normal oxygen.

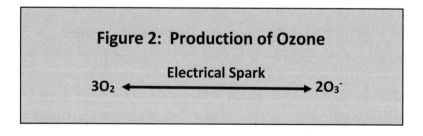

Figure 2: Production of Ozone

Electrical Spark

$$3O_2 \longleftrightarrow 2O_3^-$$

Effects of Ozone on the Human Body

Dr. Frank Shallenberger, one of the pioneers of ozone therapy in the U.S., has described many different effects ozone has on the human body.[2] He documents that ozone:

- increases oxygen delivery to tissues
- increases red blood cell membrane flexibility
- kills bacteria
- kills fungi and yeasts
- kills parasites
- kills viruses with a direct viricidal effect
- makes people feel better

Dr. Shallenberger also found that ozone stimulates:

- production of tumor necrosis factor (TNF)
- energy production in the body
- production of white blood cells
- secretion of interleukin-2, which regulates immune system functioning
- production and utilization of antioxidants

Other research shows that ozone: [3] [4] [5] [6]

- activates cellular and humoral immune systems

- activates protein synthesis

- enhances cell metabolism

- is a potent analgesic

- is the strongest naturally occurring oxidant

- is produced by immune cells

- is a more effective bactericidal agent than chlorine—it can kill bacteria 100x faster

- is an effective antibacterial agent, as demonstrated by over 100 years of medical history

- induces prostacyclin production when administered medically, which inhibits the formation of blood clots

- increases muscle oxygenation

- increases tumor oxygenation

- stimulates the proliferation of immunocomplement cells

- stimulates the synthesis of interleukins, leukotrienes, and prostaglandins

- stimulates the synthesis of immunoglobulins

Stimulating the Immune System

Ozone is an oxidative agent. Ozone is known to generate reactive oxygen species such as superoxide (O_3^-), hydroxyl radicals (OH^-), hydrogen peroxide (H_2O_2), and hypochlorous acid (HOCL). All of these substances are also produced by the soldiers of the immune system—the white blood cells—when they are fighting infections.[7] [8] In fact, during times of stress such as in an infectious state, the immune system produces many different free radicals in order to kill the offending organism and further stimulate the immune system.

Some researchers believe that ozone is produced in the body during an infectious episode, along with other oxidizing molecules listed above, in order to help the immune system fight an infection.[9]

How Does Ozone Kill Pathogens?

There are multiple ways ozone combats infections in the body. First, ozone has a direct antimicrobial effect—killing bacteria, viruses, parasites, and fungi, including yeast. Additionally, ozone has been shown to stimulate the immune system to produce antibodies that kill pathogens.[10]

Ozone also has immune regulating properties. Acting on the immune system, ozone functions as a signal that results in the production of various proteins that stimulate the immune system to recruit white blood cells to infected areas of the body to control the infection. Examples of these proteins include nuclear factor kappa B, interleukin-6 (IL-6), and tumor necrosis factor-α (TNF-α).[11] [12]

In organisms that produce spores, such as fungi, ozone has been shown to render the spores unable to reproduce due to damage to the inner membrane of the spore.[13]

To summarize, ozone can help fight infections in several ways:

- Ozone kills viruses, including Ebola and HIV

- Ozone kills bacteria

- Ozone kills parasites

- Ozone kills fungi

- Ozone kills yeast

- Ozone improves the circulation of blood

- Ozone oxygenates cells and tissues

- Ozone stimulates and supports the immune system

Ozone Kills Pathogens by Oxygenating the Body

Many bacteria, parasites, and viruses (as well as all cancers) prefer to live in an anaerobic environment. Anaerobic refers to a lack of oxygen. These anaerobic organisms will not survive in an aerobic—high oxygen—environment. Therefore, increasing an infected tissue's oxygen levels can be expected to help fight anaerobic organisms.

Ozone can be utilized to increase the release of oxygen to the tissues. As described above, ozone is created by exposing oxygen to an electrical source. The formula for ozone production is shown in Figure 3.

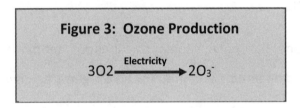

Figure 3: Ozone Production

$$3O2 \xrightarrow{\text{Electricity}} 2O_3^-$$

Ozone then rapidly combines with other oxygen molecules to re-form as the more stable, common oxygen element (O2) as shown in Figure 4.

Figure 4: Ozone into Oxygen

$$O3^- + O3^- \longrightarrow 3O2$$

Therefore, ozone therapy would be expected to increase the oxygen content of the tissues of the body, which it does.

Ozone and Bacteria

In many countries without the availability of expensive antibiotics, ozone is used to treat common infections. Ozone is inexpensive to manufacture and use. Cuba is one example of a country where ozone therapy is widely used to treat many different conditions, including infectious diseases. Cuban physicians have published a plethora of research about ozone, including articles about ozone treating viral infections as well as other illnesses including Candida (a fungal infection), burns, ulcers, and diarrhea from Giardia.

Ozone has been shown to kill both antibiotic-resistant bacteria and anaerobic (adapted for an oxygen-free environment) bacteria.[14]

My 107-Patient COVID-19 Study and Ozone Therapy

In my published study on treating COVID-19 patients (see Appendix), we provided intramuscular ozone to 36% (or 38 out of 107) of our patients. The patients who received ozone either asked for it or were recommended it because they were among the sickest patients in our practice during that time period. Of these, a single ozone injection was given to 31 (82%). Seven (18%) required more than one IM injection. Five received two ozone shots, one patient had four and another had six. The patients who required four and six injections had been ill for a longer time period (over ten days) before instituting therapy. Both recovered uneventfully.

All patients who received ozone injections fully recovered from COVID-19.

Ozone, the Immune System, and Viral Infections

In viral infections, ozone has been shown to improve both the innate and adaptive immune systems while also reducing cytokine storm. Ozone improves neutrophil counts in children with compromised phagocyte cell-mediated immunity.[15] In other words, children who have innate immune system issues respond to ozone.

Antibodies have been shown to kill pathogens by producing ozone gas.[16]

Ozone has been shown to have direct viricidal effects by disrupting the lipid envelope of a virus at sites of double bonds. When the lipid envelope is fragmented, its DNA or RNA cannot survive. SARS-CoV-2 is an enveloped virus, which would make it an excellent candidate for treatment with ozone.[17]

Furthermore, SARS-CoV-2, as well as other coronaviruses, have abundant cysteine—a thiol-containing amino acid—in their spike proteins. This thiol group contains sulfur. Cysteine can be oxidized reversibly to disulfide, which is widely understood to

155

neutralize the function of its protein/enzyme.[18] When this occurs, viral replication and function are disrupted.

Ozone and hydrogen peroxide have similar mechanisms as to how they work as antiviral, antibacterial, and anti-parasitic agents. Many of these mechanisms were described in the hydrogen peroxide chapter but bear repeating. Rowen has hypothesized that ozone is the ideal therapy for viruses. To successfully penetrate cell membranes, many viruses require membrane glycoproteins to be in the R-S-H reduced form as opposed to the oxidized—R-S-S-R— form. If virus thiol groups are oxidized, they lose infectivity.[19] Rowen states, "Creating a more 'oxidized' environment [may allow] ozone therapy...[to] assist the body in inactivating thiols in viruses in blood and tissues. SARS-CoV-2 cell entry spike proteins are particularly rich in both cysteine and tryptophan, the two most vulnerable amino acids to alteration by ozone."[20] [21] The thiol group of cysteine is easily oxidized. Effectively, it functions as an "on-off" switch. Potent oxidants, such as hydrogen peroxide or ozone, can irreversibly oxidize the thiol. Regardless, viruses have no means to self-repair even when in the disulfide oxidation state. Regarding tryptophan, it is also easily oxidized by ozone.[22] [23]

Ozone, like ascorbate (vitamin C), has been shown to increase the production of hydrogen peroxide.[24] [25] This viral redox vulnerability theory was verified with the use of ozone rapidly remitting five cases of Ebola in 2014. The Ebola virus similarly to

SARS-CoV-2 has a large quantity of cysteine in its membrane glycoproteins.[26]

Ozone, hydrogen peroxide and intravenous vitamin C all share very similar properties on how they work as viricidal agents. That is why I included all three therapies in my viral protocol—they have synergistic effects when they are given together.

COVID-19 is associated with micro thrombotic (blood clotting) events and, often, a cytokine storm of inflammation. Ozone could be particularly useful as it improves the prostacyclin:thromboxane ratio and enhances nitric oxide production.[27] Ozone has been shown to reduce production of TNF-alpha[28] as effectively as steroids do, and increases the production of the anti-inflammatory enzyme heme oxygenase-1.[29] Therefore, ozone therapy should counter the increase in thrombotic events observed in COVID-19 patients. None of our patients suffered a thrombotic event while on our therapy. Some indeed did have blood clots accompanying COVID-19 symptoms—before beginning our treatment plan. These patients improved on the protocol and the blood clots resolved.

Final Thoughts

Ozone therapy is not taught in US medical schools—at least that is my understanding after watching two children attend medical school and mentoring many other medical students and residents. In fact, when I ask the medical students and residents about ozone, they usually have a blank look on their faces as they have not heard it mentioned once during their training.

Ozone has direct viricidal effects. But, it is important to keep in mind it also has a killing effect on bacteria, parasites and yeast. It is one of the most important therapies I do in my office.

Ozone is given as a gas. It can be utilized via an IV, hyperbaric treatment, and as an intramuscular injection. Ozone can also be used in the ears as well as rectally or vaginally. The reason I used it intramuscularly in my study was because I knew it was an effective therapy from previous use and it was the safest way to administer it outside during the pandemic. I did not want COVID-19 patients coming into my office since I did not want to expose my staff.

One of the most potent ways to use ozone is a hyperbaric method known as a 10-pass treatment. In this method, we can ozonate one-third of the blood supply in approximately one hour. It is a wonderful treatment for acute infections. Robert Rowen, my mentor on ozone (and, who taught me how to do the hyperbaric treatment) has used the 10-pass therapy on acutely ill COVID-19 patients. He reported that his patients improved as they were receiving the treatment.[30]

Ozone is a very safe therapy when it is in skilled hands. To get the best results from ozone, it is important to work with a

holistic practitioner who can prescribe the best method for
ozonating your body.

[1] World Federation of Ozone Therapy's Review on Evidence Based Ozone
Therapy.. 2015. 7.
[2] Accessed 6.29.16 from :
http://www.ozonedetox.com/ozone/ozoneEffectsShallenberger.htm
[3] PNAS, 100(6):3031-4. 2003
[4] Evid. Based Complement. Alternat. Med., 1: 93–8. 2004
[5] Afr. J. Infect. Dis. (2016) 10 (1): 49– 54
[6] J Nat Sci Biol Med. 2011 Jul-Dec; 2(2): 151–153
[7] Annu. Rev. Biochm. 49:695. 1980
[8] J. Clin. Invest. 99:424-432. 1997
[9] Trends. Biochem. Sci. 29:274-78. 2004
[10] Science. Vol. 298. 12.13. 2002
[11] Allergy. 55.321 (2000)
[12] Am. J. Physiol. 280. L537 (2002)
[13] Applied Microbiology. Vol. 96, N. 5. May, 2004. 1133
[14] Bocci, V. Ozone. A New Medical Drug. Springer. 2005
[15] Díaz LJ, Sardiñas PG, Menéndez CS, et al. Immunomodulator effect of ozone
therapy in children with deficiency in immunity mediated by
phagocytes. Mediciego. 2012;18(1)
[16] Wentworth P. Evidence for Antibody-Catalyzed Ozone Formation in Bacterial
Killing and Inflammation. *Science*. 2002;298(5601):2195-2199.
doi:10.1126/science.1077642
[17] Walter LA, McGregor AJ. Sex- and Gender-specific Observations and
Implications for COVID-19. *West J Emerg Med*. 2020;21(3):507-509. Published
2020 Apr 10. doi:10.5811/westjem.2020.4.47536

[18] Brownstein, D., et al. A Novel Approach to Treating COVID-19 with
Nutritional and Oxidative Therapies. *Science, Public Health Policy, and The Law*
Volume 2:4-22 July, 2020 Clinical and Translational Research
[19] Mirazimi A, Mousavi-Jazi M, Sundqvist VA, Svensson L. Free thiol groups are
essential for infectivity of human cytomegalovirus. *J Gen Virol*. 1999;80 (Pt
11):2861-2865. doi:10.1099/0022-1317-80-11-2861
[20] Broer R, Boson B, Spaan W, Cosset FL, Corver J. Important role for the
transmembrane domain of severe acute respiratory syndrome coronavirus
spike protein during entry. *J Virol*. 2006;80(3):1302-1310.
doi:10.1128/JVI.80.3.1302-1310.2006

[21]Virender K. Sharma & Nigel J.D. Graham (2010) Oxidation of Amino Acids, Peptides and Proteins by Ozone: A Review, Ozone: Science & Engineering, 32:2, 81-90, DOI: 10.1080/01919510903510507

[22] KUNAPULI S, KHAN N, DIVAKAR N, VAIDYANATHAN C. OXIDATION OF INDOLES. Journal of the Indian Institute of Science. http://journal.library.iisc.ernet.in/index.php/iisc/article/view/3973. Published 2020.

[23] Virender, K., et al. IBID. 2010.

[24] IBID. Bocci V. *Oxygen-Ozone Therapy*. Dordrecht: Springer; 2002:1440

[25] IBID. Bocci, V. & Aldinucci, Carlo & Bianchi, L.. (2005). The use of hydrogen peroxide as a medical drug. Rivista Italiana di Ossigeno-Ozonoterapia. 4. 30-39

[26]3. Lopez L, Riffle A, Pike S, Gardner D, Hogue B (2008) Importance of conserved cysteine residues in the coronavirus envelope protein. J Virol 82: 3000-3010.

[27] Schulz S, Ninke S, Watzer B, Nüsing RM. Ozone induces synthesis of systemic prostacyclin by cyclooxygenase-2 dependent mechanism in vivo. *Biochem Pharmacol*. 2012;83(4):506-513. doi:10.1016/j.bcp.2011.11.025

[28] Zamora ZB, Borrego A, López OY, et al. Effects of ozone oxidative preconditioning on TNF-alpha release and antioxidant-prooxidant intracellular balance in mice during endotoxic shock. *Mediators Inflamm*. 2005;2005(1):16-22. doi:10.1155/MI.2005.16

[29] Pecorelli A, Bocci V, Acquaviva A, et al. NRF2 activation is involved in ozonated human serum upregulation of HO-1 in endothelial cells. *Toxicol Appl Pharmacol*. 2013;267(1):30-40. doi:10.1016/j.taap.2012.12.001

[30] Personal communication with Robert Rowen, M.D.

Chapter 9

Why Nebulizing Is Important

Why Nebulizing Is Important

Introduction

I have been recommending nebulized therapies to my patients for over 20 years. 'Nebulize' is a 19th century term derived from Latin. 'Nebula' comes from the Latin word for 'mist' and 'ize' means 'to become'. So, nebulizing refers to converting a substance to a fine mist or spray, especially for inhalation of a medicinal drug.

Nebulizers are devices that allow the user to breathe in a medication as a fine mist. Asthmatics have used nebulizers for decades. Over the years, I found nebulizing natural substances such as hydrogen peroxide, iodine, and glutathione helpful for patients ill with a variety of viral infections, including influenza-like illnesses.

COVID-19 Patients and Nebulizing

My patients who became ill with COVID-19 had much more severe lung involvement than is typically seen during influenza seasons. In COVID-19 patients, nebulizing a combination of dilute hydrogen peroxide and iodine became an essential therapy for most of them. In fact, 85% of the patients in my COVID-19 study used nebulized hydrogen peroxide and iodine successfully (see Appendix).[1]

Due to the success I saw with COVID-19 patients who nebulized hydrogen peroxide and iodine, I felt this topic deserved its own chapter.

As I stated above, I have been recommending nebulizing for viral infections and pneumonia as well as other lung conditions for over 20 years. For multiple viral illnesses, nebulizing hydrogen peroxide and iodine has proven successful over this time period. In fact, this therapy almost always improves a patient's symptoms from a variety of lung diseases including asthma, allergies, bronchitis, and even lung cancer.

Hydrogen Peroxide

The physiology and biochemistry of hydrogen peroxide was covered in more detail in Chapter 7, as well as in my book *Ozone: The Miracle Therapy*. In this Chapter, I will provide you with a summary of hydrogen peroxide's effects and refer you to the other sources for more information.

As we explored in Chapter 7, hydrogen peroxide is produced in the lungs.[2] Hydrogen peroxide is also present in exhaled air of healthy humans as well as those with lung diseases.[3] Although it is uncertain where the lungs produce hydrogen peroxide, it is thought that white blood cells in the lungs (polymorphonuclear cells—PMNs) may be producing it in order to control bacterial growth. This may explain why those with inflammatory lung diseases, as well as cigarette smokers, have been found to exhale more hydrogen peroxide than other subjects.[4]

Hydrogen peroxide is produced by the white blood cells to fight infectious organisms. Smokers, who are at an increased risk for pulmonary problems from infectious organisms, produce more hydrogen peroxide than nonsmokers.[5]

Vaporized hydrogen peroxide has been successfully utilized to control multidrug-resistant infections in a long-term acute care hospital. Although this was not the same therapy as having a human breathe in nebulized hydrogen peroxide, it shows the effectiveness of hydrogen peroxide in a vaporized form at killing a multidrug-resistant infectious organism.

Hydrogen Peroxide as an Anti-Infective Therapy

In conventional medicine, hydrogen peroxide is widely used as an anti-infective substance. It is used topically on wounds and is used in the oral cavity via gargling as well as directly applying to the gums for treating periodontitis. The US Food and Drug Administration (FDA) considers the application of 3% hydrogen peroxide to oral mucosa "acceptable".[6] One study found that the application of hydrogen peroxide to areas affected by severe periodontitis reduced the bacterial overgrowth of infected areas.[7]

Many viral illnesses, particularly influenza and influenza-like illnesses, can degenerate into dangerous lung infections such as pneumonia and respiratory failure. This has been the main cause of death in those who succumbed to COVID-19. Since hydrogen peroxide is a natural, effective antimicrobial agent, it should follow that nebulizing a dilute solution of hydrogen peroxide should aid those with pathogenic lung infections, both viral and bacterial in origin, especially if it can be applied directly to the lungs. I have over 20 years of experience using nebulized hydrogen peroxide with patients suffering from infected lungs, and even in patients without lung infections but who suffer with lung diseases such as chronic obstructive pulmonary disease and fibrosis of the lungs. My experience clearly shows that nebulized hydrogen peroxide is a positive therapy for those with lung infections.

Iodine

Iodine was covered in more detail in Chapter 6. Iodine is an essential nutrient we cannot live without. Every cell in the body requires adequate iodine levels for healthy functioning. Iodine has both direct and indirect viricidal and bactericidal properties.

As I stated in Chapter 6, It has been known for over 70 years that iodine not only has potent antiviral abilities, it also functions as a broad range antiseptic agent as well, and is still used to disinfect the skin prior to hypodermic needle insertion or surgery. In 1945 iodine was found to protect mice from becoming infected with influenza virus.[8] Also, it is important to keep in mind that iodine is needed by the immune system to provide lifelong immunity to various infectious organisms. Iodine enables the white blood cells to effectively phagocytize (engulf and destroy) foreign invaders.[9]

In my study, iodine was used in both nebulized form and as an oral supplement.[10] Researchers have also reported that nasal inhalation of iodine was found to be effective at removing pathogenic bacteria that colonize the upper airways, which are a major cause of pneumonia.[11]

Nebulizing

There are many different nebulizers on the market. They fall into three categories:

- pneumatic jet nebulizers
- ultrasonic nebulizers
- vibrating mesh nebulizers (handheld)

Pneumatic Jet Nebulizers

This is the most common type of nebulizer. It consists of a compressor, oxygen tubing, a nebulizer cup to hold the liquid being nebulized, and a mouthpiece. It is powered by plugging it into an electrical outlet. It works by having air flow rapidly through a jet. This rapid airstream allows the solution being nebulized to form a mist for inhalation. Many insurance plans cover this type of nebulizer.

Ultrasonic Nebulizers

Ultrasonic nebulizers use a crystal transducer that creates a high frequency vibration in the liquid being nebulized. This creates a mist that can be inhaled. They are quieter than jet nebulizers.

Portable Handheld Mesh Nebulizers

These nebulizers sometimes run on batteries. They are usually handheld units. They work by vibrating an element in order to move liquid through a fine mesh to produce an aerosol.

Which Type of Nebulizer Should You Use?

I do not recommend using handheld battery-operated nebulizers. They simply do not have enough power to supply a therapeutic dose of a treatment to the lungs. During the COVID-19 crisis, I had two patients who failed to improve while using a handheld nebulizer to nebulize hydrogen peroxide and iodine. When they changed to a pneumatic jet nebulizer unit, they started their path to overcoming COVID-19.

Jet nebulizers are the least expensive nebulizers. They can be purchased for around $40-60. I find little reason to spend much more on a nebulizer.

How To Use a Nebulizer

A jet nebulizer is extremely easy to use. They are portable and require an electrical outlet for power.

The first step is to unpack the equipment and place the elements on a countertop near an electrical outlet. Wash your hands with soap and water, as you want to keep the nebulizer clean between uses. Assembly is simple: First, insert the tubing into the compressor. Next, put the solution into the cup. Attach the mouthpiece to the cup. Now, place the other end of the tubing connected to the compressor into the port below the cup, which contains the solution being nebulized. A picture of a nebulizer is shown below.

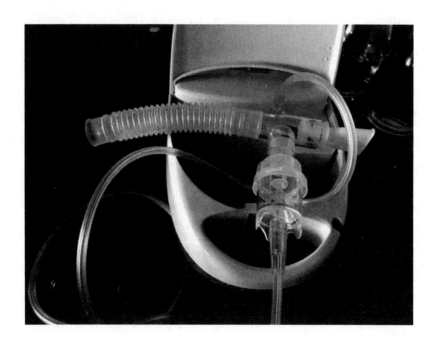

Now you are ready to use the nebulizer. Plug it into the

outlet and turn it on. A hissing sound should be heard as the air is bubbling the solution in the cup. A thin mist should be seen exiting from the end of the mouthpiece. Simply breathe in the solution until the fine mist goes away. Once done, disassemble the cup and mouthpiece and thoroughly clean them. A separate mouthpiece and cup should be used for each person using the nebulizer.

Again, I have found handheld nebulizers ineffective for providing enough nebulized solution to the lungs in order to help overcome an infectious process. I recommend using a desktop nebulizer over a handheld one. My experience has shown that a pneumatic jet nebulizer provides the proper power to effectively nebulize a solution.

Nebulized Hydrogen Peroxide and Iodine

At my office, we mix up a solution of sterile, normal saline and hydrogen peroxide for our patients to use. We use a bag of 250 cc of sterile, normal saline solution and sterilely inject 3 cc of 3% food grade hydrogen peroxide into the bag. That provides for a final concentration of 0.04% hydrogen peroxide. In my experience, this is the ideal hydrogen peroxide mixture to nebulize. This bag is kept refrigerated and can last for three months if kept cold.

Nebulizing has multiple positive effects on the lungs. It helps to moisturize the lungs, which aids in their ability to detoxify. Even just nebulizing sterile, normal saline solution has been shown to have positive effects in infants with viral bronchiolitis.[12]

My patients are instructed to draw off 3 cc of the dilute hydrogen peroxide/saline mixture and place it in the nebulizer cup. Then, one drop of 5% Lugol's solution is added to the cup. The combined hydrogen peroxide/iodine mixture is nebulized until the mist is gone.

At the first sign of an illness such as a sore throat, cough, runny nose or fever, I instruct my patients to begin nebulizing. During an acute illness, I have my patients nebulize once every waking hour as described above. They can then decrease the frequency as they are feeling better.

During the COVID-19 crises, my partners and I would treat sick patients outside the office, in the parking lot. After treatment, we would nebulize with the hydrogen peroxide/iodine mixture to kill any pathogens that may have colonized our throat or nasal cavities. All through the COVID-19 crisis, I would nebulize after work and after going into a store, or when I was out in public. This was during the height of the crisis.

Final Thoughts

My experience has clearly shown that nebulizing hydrogen peroxide and iodine, in the quantities described above, provides satisfying results for patients suffering from upper respiratory and other influenza-like illnesses, including COVID-19. The earlier one starts nebulizing when an illness strikes, the better it works.

I have not witnessed any side effects from nebulizing the hydrogen peroxide/iodine mixture described in this chapter. Rarely, the addition of one drop of 5% Lugol's iodine causes a drying, irritating feeling in the throat. If that is the case, I just have the patient nebulize the dilute hydrogen peroxide solution without iodine. These patients also received positive benefits.

There is concern that nebulizing can spread contagious illnesses. Since both the hydrogen peroxide and iodine in the mixture have direct anti-viral and bactericidal properties, it would seem this risk is low. However, I cannot quote a study verifying this point. Therefore, if one is ill with a contagious illness, it is best to nebulize outside.

Nebulizing should not be done without a doctor's supervision. I am providing instructions here with the caveat that you should only undertake this therapy under a doctor's supervision.

[1] Brownstein, D, *et al*. A Novel Approach to Treating COVID-19 Using Nutritional and Oxidative Therapies.*Science, Public Health Policy, and The Law*. Volume 2;July, 2020. P, 4-22.

[2] Rysz J, Stolarek RA, Luczynski R, *et al*. Increased hydrogen peroxide concentration in the exhaled breath condensate of stable COPD patients after nebulized N-acetylcysteine . Pulm Pharmacol Ther., 20(3):281-289, 2007.

[3] Journal of Biological Chemistry Volume 258, Issue 6, 1983, Pages 3628-3631

[4] Chest, 96 (1989), pp. 606–612

[5] Greening, A.P., *et al*.; Extracellular Release of Hydrogen Peroxide by Human Alveolar Macrophages: The Relationship to Cigarette Smoking and Lower Respiratory Tract Infections. *Clin Sci (Lond)* 1 December 1983; 65 (6): 661–664. doi: https://doi.org/10.1042/cs0650661

[6] Food and Drug Administration. Oral health care drug products for over-the-counter human use; Antigingivitis/antiplaque drug products; Establishment of a monograph. *Fed. Regist.* **68**, 32232–32286 (2003).

[7] Kanno, T., *et al*. Adjunctive antimicrobial chemotherapy based on hydrogen peroxide photolysis for non-surgical treatment of moderate to severe periodontitis: a randomized controlled trial. *Sci Rep* **7,** 12247 (2017). https://doi.org/10.1038/s41598-017-12514-0.

[8] Burnet, FM, Holden, HF, and Stone, JD. Action of iodine vapour on influenza virus in droplet suspension. *Aust J Sci*. 1945;7:125.

[9]Zel'tser ME. Vliianie khronicheskogo defitsita ĭoda v ratsione na razvitie infektsionnogo protsessa [Effect of a chronic iodine deficit in the ration on the development of the infectious process]. *Zh Mikrobiol Epidemiol Immunobiol*. 1975;0(9):116-119.

[10] IBID. Brownstein, D., *et al*. 2020

[11] Kawana A, Kudo K. *Kansenshogaku Zasshi*. 1999;73(5):429-436. doi:10.11150/kansenshogakuzasshi1970.73.429

[12]Kuzik, B, *et al*. Nebulized Hypertonic Saline in the Treatment of Viral Bronchiolitis in Infants. The Journal of Pediatrics. September, 2007. Vol. 151. Issue 3, p. 266-270

Chapter 10

Other Therapies

Other Therapies

Introduction

My 25-year, clinically tested protocol for supporting the immune system during times of viral illness consists of using oral vitamins A, C, D and iodine as well as nebulized hydrogen peroxide.[1] If the situation warrants further care, intravenous doses of vitamin C, hydrogen peroxide and either IV or intramuscular injections of ozone have proven effective. My partners and I found,

177

during the COVID-19 crisis, that our therapy worked just as it worked over the last 25 years during the influenza season.

However, other therapies have been touted as effective against SARS-CoV-2 / COVID-19. This chapter will review some of those other treatments.

Hydroxychloroquine

Hydroxychloroquine was originally derived from the cinchona tree and the ancient Incas utilized it to combat fevers. It was imported to Europe in 1630 by Spanish doctors or Jesuit priests, who noted its fever-lowering abilities. In the 1800s, French doctors began using it for malaria-induced fevers. The British used the drug in British colonies located in malaria-infested areas. U.S. doctors began using hydroxychloroquine in the 20th century to treat autoimmune arthritic diseases such as Lupus and rheumatoid arthritis.

In March 2020, President Trump promoted the use of hydroxychloroquine as a preventive and treatment for SARS-CoV-2, stating: "I sure as hell think we ought to give it a try." Later, he tweeted the use of hydroxychloroquine with azithromycin, an antibiotic, could be "...one of the biggest game-changers in the history of medicine." A few days later, Trump tweeted again about hydroxychloroquine, stating, "...there are some very strong, powerful signs..." of its potential as a COVID-19 therapy." [2]

This started a political firestorm, with President Trump's own health advisors urging caution with the use of hydroxychloroquine, stating that there is only anecdotal evidence of its effectiveness with COVID-19. The mainstream news media took the position that hydroxychloroquine was dangerous and not effective for treating a viral infection, particularly COVID-19.

I have used hydroxychloroquine for treating autoimmune and parasitic infections for many years. When used appropriately, it is very safe and it is not dangerous. I have not utilized it for treating viral infections.

Didier Raoult, M.D., a French virologist, touted the use of hydroxychloroquine for treating patients suffering from COVID-19. Similarly, Vladimir Zelenko, M.D., a family practitioner from Monroe, New York, utilized a five-day therapy consisting of hydroxychloroquine (200 mg twice per day), azithromycin (500 mg once per day) and zinc sulfate (220 mg once per day). Dr. Zelenko reported treating approximately 500 patients and reported zero deaths, hospitalizations or intubations.

It is theorized that hydroxychloroquine helps zinc enter a cell. Zinc can slow viral replication inside a cell. The antibiotic (azithromycin) was utilized to prevent a secondary bacterial infection. The low-dose hydroxychloroquine therapy utilized by Dr. Zelenko is similar to the doses I have prescribed over the years.

Multiple studies on the use of hydroxychloroquine and COVID-19 were completed with extremely ill hospitalized COVID-19 patients as subjects. These studies found no positive effects with the use of hydroxychloroquine. An outpatient study published in *The New England Journal of Medicine* that was randomized, double-blind, and placebo-controlled, reported no difference in COVID-19 symptoms between a control group and a COVID-19-exposed group treated with hydroxychloroquine.[3] It is notable that neither zinc nor azithromycin was used in this study.

A study from Henry Ford Health System found treatment with hydroxychloroquine cut the death rate by 50% in patients hospitalized with COVID-19.[4] The study found 13% of those treated with hydroxychloroquine alone died compared to 26.4% not treated with hydroxychloroquine. None of the patients suffered serious heart problems.

Final Thoughts: Hydroxychloroquine

Does hydroxychloroquine work for COVID-19 and perhaps other viral infections? Unfortunately, I cannot give you a straight "yes" or "no" since I have no experience with it. It is a shame that the use of hydroxychloroquine has been so politicized. So far, I think there are enough negative studies to question the effectiveness of hydroxychloroquine in relation to COVID-19. However, Dr. Zelenko's accounts of his use of the drug and the Henry Ford Health System study are compelling. Although the drug is safe at low doses, there are potential serious side effects when large doses are used.

Would I take hydroxychloroquine for COVID-19? No. I would take my protocol! Do I think hydroxychloroquine should be limited for use? No way! Competent physicians should be able to use a drug off-label to treat their patients to the best of their abilities.

Remdesivir

Remdesivir is an antiviral medication that was synthesized for use in Ebola infection. In the case of Ebola, Remdesivir failed. Initial studies of Remdesivir with treating COVID-19 patients found it reduced the length of hospitalization by four days—15 days in the control group versus 11 days in the treatment group. When this study was released, the FDA quickly approved Remdesivir for use in hospitalized COVID-19 patients.[5]

The drug works by inhibiting viral RNA synthesis. It was found to have activity against SARS-CoV, MERS CoV, and SARS CoV-2 in cell culture (in vitro) as well as in animal models.

Adverse side effects can occur with Remdesivir. A randomized clinical trial studying adults with severe COVID-19 found that 74% treated with Remdesivir had an adverse event. Serious adverse events were found in 35%. A serious adverse event is defined as:[6]

- a life-threatening event

- death

- inpatient hospitalization or prolongation of existing hospitalization

- a persistent or significant incapacity or substantial disruption of the ability to conduct normal life functions

- a congenital anomaly/birth defect

- a medical or surgical intervention to prevent death, a life-threatening event, hospitalization, disability, or congenital anomaly.

A cohort of 53 hospitalized patients treated with Remdesivir reported 60% of those treated suffered adverse effects such as increased liver enzymes, diarrhea, rash, renal impairment, and hypotension. Serious adverse effects were reported in 23%, which included: multiple organ dysfunction syndrome, septic shock, acute kidney injury, and hypotension.

The cost of Remdesivir is not for the faint of heart. Depending on the insurance status, the cost of a trial of Remdesivir will be from $2340 to $3,120.

Final Thoughts: Remdesivir

As of June 29, 2020, the US Department of Health and Human Services allocated 500,000 treatment courses of Remdesivir through September. If I take the median cost of Remdesivir--$2,730–that comes out to a grand total cost to U.S. taxpayers of $1,365,000,000. Keep in mind: this price tag is not for a cure for COVID-19; it's for several fewer days in the hospital, on average.

What a deal.

After looking at the adverse effects, not only would I not take this medication, I would counsel my patients to avoid it. The adverse effects are not worth a few less hospital days and no mortality benefit.

Diet, Hydration and Exercise

I cannot overstate the importance of eating a healthy diet. This means adopting a healthy lifestyle *before* you become ill with a viral or any other illness. The number one reason Americans are suffering from such serious health problems, including COVID-19, is because they generally eat a poor diet.

An unhealthy diet is one that contains too much sugar as well as too much refined flour, salt, and oils. Refined foods are deficient in basic vitamins, minerals and fats, and contain toxic byproducts as well. The consequence of eating an unhealthy diet is weight gain and a drop in energy levels. Furthermore, a poor diet predisposes one to getting diabetes, hypertension, heart disease, cancer, autoimmune illnesses, and a host of other chronic conditions as well as increased susceptibility to infectious agents such as viruses.

A healthy diet consists of eating organic food free of pesticides, insecticides and synthetic hormones. This diet should include healthy sources of fruits, vegetables, nuts, beans, and seeds. A healthy diet can include animal products if the animal food source is raised appropriately, free of toxic chemicals and hormones.

The next part of a healthy diet consists of maintaining adequate hydration. Avoid dehydration at all times—especially if you think you may become ill with any infectious organism. Simply put: You must always drink an adequate amount of water. How much water should you drink? Take you weight in pounds, divide that number by 2. The resulting number is the minimum amount of water to drink in ounces per day.

Lastly, I cannot overemphasize the importance of regular exercise. Exercise helps every known condition. Keeping your body in shape will help it in a time of infection or when your body is confronted with any stressful situation. Your innate and adaptive immune systems will be more able to properly respond and overcome a foreign pathogen if it is in optimal shape *before* the illness starts. Keep in mind with COVID-19, a major risk factor for a poor outcome was being overweight.

Final Thoughts:
Diet, Hydration and Exercise

Many people feel overwhelmed by trying to eat a healthy diet. There is nothing to be overwhelmed by. It just takes a little education and elbow grease and a healthy diet can be part of your daily regimen. Although a long discussion on a healthy diet is beyond the scope of this book, I have written a book, *The Guide to Healthy Eating*, which can help you find your way.

Sweating

Sweating is an important function in the body. Sweating serves many purposes—it is a mode for the body to release toxins. I have been detoxifying my patients from heavy metals, and I can assure you that those who do not sweat have a much more difficult time reducing their toxic load.

For more than two decades, I have encouraged my patients to sweat on a regular basis. Of course, the best way to sweat is to exercise. However, benefits from sweating can also occur from a sauna or a hot tub.

For patients who cannot sweat, I encourage them to start slowly with a hot Epsom salt bath or a sauna. Putting 3% hydrogen peroxide on the skin before a bath or sauna can help stimulate the sweat glands.

In the case of an acute infection with fever, sweating is an especially important body function. It is a way for the body to release toxic particles and a way to cool itself down. One study found glycoproteins in the skin were able to bind microbial agents and remove them via sweating.[7]

At the first sign of an illness, I suggest heating the body with either an Epsom salt bath, taking a sauna or getting in a hot tub. The ability to sweat can aid your recovery from an infectious process. In the case of coronavirus, the World Health Organization reported that temperatures over 132°F can kill coronavirus.[8] Therefore, sitting in a sauna over 132°F may help in SARS-CoV-2 infections.

Fever

A fever is the body's way of fighting an infection. We have been conditioned to avoid a fever. Commercials extol the virtue of taking over-the-counter medications such as acetaminophen or ibuprofen to control a fever. In most cases, that is the last thing you want to do. In fact, the increase of the core temperature serves many positive functions in the body.

A fever is a signal to the immune system that something is wrong in the body. When a fever is present, the immune system speeds up the delivery of immune cells to areas of infection or inflammation. A fever stimulates the production of two molecules that help immune cells (T cells) migrate from the bloodstream to the lymph nodes near an infection. This allows them to move to the problem areas of the body and start the process of neutralizing the offending organism.

In the case of an infectious process, as long as the fever is below 103°F, I do not recommend using an anti-fever medication. as that will blunt the immune system's response. Body temperatures higher than 103°F can lead to a seizure.

Furthermore, acetaminophen should be avoided in all infectious illnesses as it depletes the body of an important antioxidant glutathione. Acetaminophen should only be used as a last resort.

Ibuprofen is also associated with adverse effects. Its use is associated with an increased risk of bleeding and a decrease in blood flow to the kidneys. The use of Ibuprofen and other non-steroidal anti-inflammatory drugs (NSAIDs) is one of the most common causes of kidney failure in the US.

The best fever control is to use a tepid bath to cool the body off when needed. I have found good success with using Epsom salt/hydrogen peroxide baths. Simply put two cups of Epsom salts and two cups of 3% over-the-counter hydrogen peroxide into the tub.

Final Thoughts: Fever

Avoid taking acetaminophen or ibuprofen-like drugs except as a last resort. Neither of these medications is benign, and they inhibit the immune system's ability to fight against a viral infection.

It is best to work with a holistic doctor who can give you safer options when trying to mitigate a fever.

Zinc

As described earlier in this chapter, Dr. Zelenko's protocol for treating COVID-19 patients was to use zinc in combination with hydroxychloroquine and azithromycin.

Zinc is an essential mineral we cannot live without. Zinc has been found to inhibit two proteins involved in the replication of the original SARS-CoV (the first coronavirus infection that spread from China, 18 years ago). These proteins are known as the 3CL protease and the papain-like protease-2. Keep in mind that SARS-CoV and SARS-CoV-2 are 87% identical when looking at protein structure. Zinc was shown to bind to the sulfur moiety found in the amino acid cysteine. Once bound, zinc inhibits these proteins.[9] [10]

Zinc does not possess viricidal activity to coronavirus. It may work by enhancing the cell's innate ability to inhibit the virus from replicating inside the cell. Zinc lozenges may help if used early in a viral illness, as the added zinc can help prevent the replication of viruses that bind to the throat.

Final Thoughts: Zinc

I have been checking zinc levels in my patients for over two decades. Approximately 40% of my patients presented with low zinc levels. I think it is essential to have optimal zinc levels *BEFORE* you become ill with any infection. As for using zinc at the start of an illness like COVID-19, I am ambivalent. I do not think a couple days of zinc lozenges or supplements would hurt anyone. However, zinc was not part of my protocol and I did not find the need for it. Perhaps it is because my patients have already been checked for their zinc status and appropriately supplemented when they need it.

Zinc supplementation can cause problems with copper levels. Copper is an essential nutrient for the human body, and I have found many patients have copper deficiencies. Supplementing zinc can cause copper levels to lower. Studies have found copper is very toxic to SARS-CoV.[11] The last thing you want to do is become copper deficient in times of an acute viral infection. Therefore, I do not recommend using zinc unless you have a zinc deficiency.

It is best to work with a holistic health care provider who can check all your mineral levels, copper and zinc included, and appropriately recommend supplementation on the basis of test results.

Melatonin

Melatonin is a natural substance produced in the body. It is best known as a 'sleeping' agent, as its production in the brain, specifically the pineal gland, rises at night. Melatonin pills are sold in most health food stores and pharmacies as a sleep aid.

However, melatonin is also produced, in large quantities, in the mitochondria—the powerhouse of the cells where energy molecules are produced. Melatonin has been shown to exist in every cell in the human body and in all living organisms, from bacteria to humans.

Melatonin is a potent free radical scavenger and antioxidant.[12] It provides protection against oxidative stress. Studies have found that both melatonin produced in the body and melatonin taken as a supplement protect against oxidative stress.[13] Melatonin has greater antioxidant activity than vitamins C and E, as well as glutathione.[14] [15]

Many viral and bacterial infections can cause an elevated inflammatory response known as cytokine storm. Antioxidants are needed by the body to counter viral-induced or bacterial-induced cytokine storm. Melatonin can be utilized for this purpose.

Macrophages are white blood cells that can engulf and destroy foreign invaders. When this destruction process occurs, oxidative stress is accelerated. Melatonin can be produced in the macrophage mitochondria. Ensuring adequate melatonin levels in the entire body and in the macrophages can minimize the chance that inflammation spirals out of control leading to cytokine storm.

Final Thoughts: Melatonin

I have utilized melatonin in my practice for well over two decades. It has provided good results to help people suffering from sleep disorders and fatigue issues. In the case of a viral infection, I think melatonin can be safely used and may provide benefit in preventing cytokine storm. The only side effects from melatonin are, if used at bedtime, next-day drowsiness or nightmares. These side effects are uncommon.

I have prescribed melatonin at dosages ranging from ½mg to 100mg per day. Your holistically minded doctor can help you with the proper dose for your situation.

Glutathione

A second-year medical student at Sophie Davis/CUNY School of Medicine was reported to have cured his mother's COVID-19 respiratory distress with 2,000 mg of glutathione. The story in the *New York Post* article stated, "After one 2,000-milligram dose, the family witnessed a miracle." Within the hour, her breathing and wellbeing dramatically improved. She took glutathione for five days and never had a recurrence of her breathing issues. The patient was also treated with zinc, alpha lipoic acid, and N- acetyl cysteine as well as vitamin C. Two case reports published in the journal, *Respiratory Medicine Case Reports* found similar findings with glutathione supplementation.[16]

The author of these case reports hypothesized that glutathione helps to reduce pro-inflammatory cytokines (TNF-α, IL-6, and IL-8) associated with cytokine storm. Glutathione is the most abundant antioxidant in the airways' epithelial lining fluid, and protects against oxidative stress.

Final Thoughts: Glutathione

Maintaining optimal glutathione levels in times of oxidative stress such as an acute viral infection will only provide benefits. Vitamin C helps to maintain optimal, reduced glutathione levels. Although glutathione supplementation was not in my protocol, I can appreciate the benefits of taking it. I may have indirectly helped my patients maintain optimal glutathione levels by supplementing with large doses of vitamin C.

Final Thoughts

Viral infections are far too common. When the immune system is in poor shape, it cannot respond appropriately to a viral infection and this can lead to serious complications. In the US, far too many people die from influenza-like illnesses. Having an intact and well-supported immune system can help the body overcome a viral infection.

When we do not let politics in the way, science should be able to dictate which therapies are effective and those that are ineffective for treating a viral illness. The information in this chapter and this book should help you make good health care choices when you are confronted with a viral illness.

[1] Brownstein, D, *et al*. A Novel Approach to Treating COVID-19 Using Nutritional and Oxidative Therapies.*Science, Public Health Policy, and The Law*. Volume 2;July, 2020. P, 4-22

[2] Accessed 7.23.20 from: https://www.theguardian.com/science/2020/apr/06/coronavirus-cure-fact-check-hydroxychloroquine-trump

[3] **A Randomized Trial of Hydroxychloroquine as Postexposure Prophylaxis for Covid-19**. *New England Journal of Medicine*, 2020; DOI: 10.1056/NEJMoa2016638

[4] Arshad, S, et al. Treatment with hydroxychloroquine, azithromycin, and combination in patients hospitalized with COVID-19. Int. J. of Infectious Diseases. 97.2020.

[5] https://www.fda.gov/media/137564/download?fbclid=IwAR2RhQ70iiaVTR6KII VenIC80GKpZpy3UuVMJyIgtlDf-fn6pi1H1BPM0QA

[6] Accessed 7.23.20. https://www.drugs.com/sfx/remdesivir-side-effects.html

[7] Robyn A Peterson, Audrey Gueniche, Ségolène Adam de Beaumais, Lionel Breton, Maria Dalko-Csiba, Nicolle H Packer, Sweating the small stuff: Glycoproteins in human sweat and their unexplored potential for microbial adhesion, *Glycobiology*, Volume 26, Issue 3, March 2016, Pages 218–229, https://doi.org/10.1093/glycob/cwv102

[8] Accessed 7.24.20 from: https://www.who.int/csr/sars/survival_2003_05_04/en/

[9] John, T.A., et al. Evaluation of metal-conjugated compounds as inhibitors of 3cl protease of SARS-CoV. FEBS Letters. 574.(2004):116-120.

[10] Yu-San Han, et al. Papain-Like Protease 2 (PLP2) from Severe Acute Respiratory Syndrome Coronavirus (SARS-CoV): Expression, Purification, Characterization, and Inhibition. Biochemistry. 2005:44:10349-10359

[11] Han J, Chen L, Duan SM, et al. Efficient and quick inactivation of SARS coronavirus and other microbes exposed to the surfaces of some metal catalysts. *Biomed Environ Sci*. 2005;18(3):176-180.

[12] Tan DX, Manchester LC, Liu X, Rosales-Corral SA, Acuna-Castroviejo D, Reiter RJ. Mitochondria and chloroplasts as the original sites of melatonin synthesis: a hypothesis related to melatonin's primary function and evolution in eukaryotes. *J Pineal Res*. 2013;54(2):127-138. doi:10.1111/jpi.12026

[13] Tan, DX. IBID. 2013.

[14] Yimaz, T., et al. The protective effects of melatonin, vitamin E, octreolide on retinal edema during ischemia-reperfusion in the guinea pig retina. Eur. J. Opth. 2002;12:443-449

[15] Sonmez, MF, Narin, F, Akkus, D, et al. Melatonin and vitamin C ameliorate alcohol-induced oxidative stress and eNOS expression in rat kidney. Ren Fail 2012; 34:480–486

[16] Horowitz, R, et al. Case Reprot: Efficacy of glutathione therapy in relieving dyspnea associated with COVID-19 pneumonia: A report of 2 cases. Vol. 30, 2020.101063. https://doi.org/10.1016/j.rmcr.2020.101063

Chapter 11

Vaccination

Vaccination

Introduction

As I write this book, America is still in the grips of the COVID-19 pandemic. There is a "warp-speed" vaccination race to see which Big Pharma company can bring to market the first vaccine for SARS-CoV-2. At the time of this writing, the US Government has spent over $9,000,000,000 in advance with the hope that a safe and effective coronavirus vaccine will be released by the end of 2020. I can only imagine what the final cost will be.

There are several different approaches to a coronavirus vaccine. Each company is using pieces of the coronavirus—

especially the coronavirus spike proteins—to stimulate the immune system to produce antibodies against SARS-CoV-2.

The vaccine candidates are based on new technologies that have not been tried before. I hope that we develop a safe and effective vaccine for SARS-CoV-2. However, a speedy process that omits many safety steps from previous vaccine trials may prove to be problematic. Time will tell.

The vaccine against influenza has been around for nearly 100 years. The virus that causes influenza mutates every year, therefore the flu vaccine is recommended on an annual basis. Coronavirus has also been shown to mutate frequently. SARS-CoV-2 is a type of coronavirus. Although the vaccines in development to prevent its infection are new, there is every reason to believe that the effectiveness of a coronavirus vaccine will mirror the influenza vaccine. That is not good news as the flu vaccine is woefully ineffective for the vast majority of the population.

Different Types of Vaccines

There are many different types of vaccines currently in the marketplace. This section will review the different vaccine types. Some illnesses such as polio or influenza have multiple vaccine modalities available. That will be explained below.

Live Vaccines

Live vaccines use a weakened—referred to as 'attenuated'—form of the pathogen that causes disease. This type of vaccine is designed to promote an antibody response by the immune system that allows the pathogen to be neutralized and removed.

Examples of live virus vaccines include:

- Chickenpox
- Influenza
- Measles
- Mumps
- Rotavirus
- Yellow fever

Since live virus vaccines more closely mimic the natural infections they are intended to prevent, they tend to create a longer-lasting immune response and require fewer doses as compared to other types of vaccines. Some live virus vaccines, such as measles and chickenpox, are more effective in preventing infection from the pathogenic organisms. Others are not so effective, such as vaccines for influenza (more about this below) and mumps.

One concern for a live virus vaccine is that the virus can be transmitted to a person who has a compromised immune system. In other words, the live virus vaccine has the potential to cause the disease it is supposed to immunize against. This adverse effect has been reported in the medical literature. Live virus vaccines need extensive safety testing to prevent this from happening.

Inactivated Vaccines

Inactivated vaccines use a killed or inactive version of the pathogenic organism that causes an illness. This type of vaccine will not transmit the germ from person to person.

An inactivated vaccine is designed to provoke an immune response against the organism to prevent an infection. Inactivated vaccines do not provide as strong an immune response, nor one that lasts as long as live virus vaccines. Therefore, to provide for long-term immunity, booster doses are often needed for inactivated vaccines.

Examples of inactivated vaccines include:

- Hepatitis A
- Influenza
- Pertussis
- Polio (injection only)
- Rabies

Subunit, Recombinant, Polysaccharide, and Conjugate Vaccines

These types of vaccines use specific pieces of the organism such as a protein, sugar, or outer shell to stimulate the immune system to produce antibodies against the specific pathogen. Booster does of these types of vaccines are often needed as they do not often provide long-lasting protection. Each of the vaccines listed below require multiple doses.

Examples of these types of vaccines include:

- Hepatitis B
- HiB (Haemophilus influenzae type b)
- HPV (Human Papillomavirus)
- Meningococcal disease
- Pneumococcal disease
- Shingles

Toxoid Vaccines

Toxoid vaccines use a toxin produced by the organism that causes a disease. This is utilized in order to stimulate the immune system to produce antibodies against the toxin produced. Booster doses of toxoid vaccines are needed as they do not produce long-term immunity.

Examples of toxoid vaccines include:

- Diphtheria
- Tetanus

Genetically Engineered Vaccines

This type of vaccine uses genetically engineered RNA or DNA which are contained in the pathogenic organism. Once injected, this should stimulate the immune system to produce an antibody against the offending organism. At present, there are no genetically engineered vaccines in use. Some SARS-CoV-2 vaccines are the first to use this technology.

Vaccination for Influenza and SARS-CoV-2

One of the major focuses of the "warp-speed" SARS-CoV-2 vaccine development project was to protect older people who are at an increased risk for mortality from all influenza-like illnesses such as SARS-CoV-2. In fact, the elderly have suffered a tremendous increase in mortality from SARS-CoV-2, just as they do from other influenza-like illnesses. Similarly, the influenza vaccine was originally designed to protect the most vulnerable—the elderly. What is rarely acknowledged by Big Pharma and the powers-that-be is that the annual influenza vaccine is virtually useless in the elderly. It is a fact that older people do not respond to any vaccine as well as younger populations. It does not take a great intellect to predict a similar outcome with the coronavirus vaccines currently in development at the time of this writing.

Influenza Vaccine for All

Some of the information from this section is taken from my newsletter, *Dr. Brownstein's Natural Way to Health*.

The Centers for Disease Control and Prevention (CDC) begins its mission statement: "As the nation's health protection agency, CDC saves lives and protects people from health threats." Regarding influenza viruses, the viruses that cause the flu, the CDC states, "Influenza viruses typically circulate in the United States annually, most commonly from late fall through early spring. Most persons who contract influenza will recover without sequelae. However, influenza can cause serious illness, hospitalization, and death, particularly among older adults, young children, pregnant women, and those with certain chronic medical conditions. Routine annual influenza vaccination for all persons aged ≥6 months who do not have contraindications has been recommended by the CDC and CDC's Advisory Committee on Immunization Practices (ACIP) since 2010"[1]

Since the CDC has been recommending the flu vaccine for nearly all Americans since 2010, we should be seeing a decline in the number of deaths from the flu if the influenza vaccine is effective. In fact, the number of deaths from influenza has not changed much in nearly 40 years.

History of the Influenza Vaccine

Let us look at the history of influenza and the flu vaccine. The first influenza pandemic occurred in 1580. Since that time, there have been numerous reports of flu pandemics. An influenza pandemic is an epidemic of the influenza virus that affects a significant portion of the worldwide population.

Pandemics can occur when a new strain of the influenza virus is transmitted to humans from a different animal species. Bats, birds, chickens, ducks and geese are known to harbor and spread influenza. In fact, influenza and influenza-like illnesses only became a problem to humans when we domesticated wild animals. COVID-19 is thought to have transferred infection to humans via a bat virus that was under study.

Most of us are familiar with the symptoms of the flu. Influenza is a viral infection that attacks the respiratory system. This includes the nose, throat, bronchial tubes, and lungs. A patient suffering from influenza typically has a runny nose, cough, and fever. Other symptoms include headache, fatigue, and congestion.

By far, most cases of the flu are self-limiting, lasting a few days to a week. Infrequently, influenza can lead to severe complications such as respiratory failure, pneumonia, and death. However, severe complications from the flu, for the vast majority, are rare.

We are told by our government, doctors, the media, and of course the Big Pharma cartel that the best way to prevent getting the flu is to get the flu vaccine. Furthermore, the powers-that-be assure us that taking the flu vaccine will prevent severe complications from the flu. Finally, they state that the flu vaccine is innocuous—everybody from children six months old to the elderly would benefit from getting the flu vaccine.

The powers-that-be should talk to Mitchell.

Mitchell is a 31-year-old pharmaceutical sales representative. Mitchell was in great shape as he worked out daily. "About five years ago, I was told by my doctor to get the flu vaccine. I have not received a vaccine since my childhood. I told the doctor that I never got the flu in my life. The doctor told me that was irrelevant, as everybody needs the flu vaccine. I did not question him at all. That was the biggest mistake I made," he said.

Mitchell was given the flu vaccine by his doctor, and that night began to feel ill. The next day, he came down with a high fever—his temperature climbed to 104°F. Mitchell's fever lasted four days. Then he began to get other symptoms. He stated, "My bones began to ache. Not a regular ache, but a deep, thick aching. I could barely get out of bed. I was taking 600mg of ibuprofen four times a day just to be able to move. Next, all my joints began aching. I felt like I turned into an old man, instantly."

Mitchell missed two weeks of work. When he went back to his physician, Mitchell was told the vaccine had nothing to do with his symptoms. Mitchell was incredulous. "Within a few hours of that shot, I began to feel sick. I knew it was the flu shot and I think he knew it was. He just wasn't going to admit it," Mitchell said.

I saw Mitchell four months after the illness began. During this time, he saw a neurologist who diagnosed Mitchell with fibromyalgia. The neurologist, to his credit, told Mitchell that his symptoms might have been caused by the flu vaccine, but there was no treatment available. At this point, Mitchell could not work out and was thinking of taking a leave of absence from work. Mitchell was fatigued and suffering from constant muscle aches and pains.

I told Mitchell I have seen other patients affected similarly by vaccines—though certainly not the majority of vaccine recipients. I treated Mitchell with a combination of vitamins and minerals (vitamin C, Vitamin B12 injections and a liver detoxification powder called Total Liver Care) to aid his detoxification pathways. I also had Mitchell undergo four nutritional intravenous treatments—Meyer's IV's. A Meyer's IV is *an intravenous nutrient cocktail given as a fast push. The Meyer's IV contains vitamin C, magnesium, B-vitamins, and minerals, all at high doses.*

Through applied kinesiology testing, I found Mitchell's energetic system was still negatively reacting to the flu vaccine. I treated Mitchell with NAET (Nambudripod's Allergy Elimination Technique), an acupressure treatment designed to treat allergies and electrical imbalances in the body. Within one month, Mitchell felt much better. "After the treatments, I was able to begin to work out," he said, "but more importantly, I felt like my old self. The muscle aches and pains went away. My wife told me that it was nice to have her husband back."

If you believe the media, most physicians, the AMA and nearly every other medical organization in the world, everybody needs to be vaccinated for the flu. In fact, the Center for Disease Control's new recommendations state, "...everyone six months and older should get a flu vaccine each year starting with the 2010-2011 influenza season. Starting in 2010, all children six months through eight years of age are recommended to receive two doses of the flu vaccine."

You would logically assume that the CDC is looking at scientific research to conclude that everybody needs the flu vaccine. Let us take a close look at the research, then you make the decision whether to follow the CDC's advice.

The CDC, Influenza Vaccination, and Facts

The CDC recommends all children aged six months and older should get the flu vaccine. Again, for the CDC to recommend that nearly everyone in the country receive a flu vaccine on an annual basis, there should be good data showing the vaccine is effective for the vast majority of the population. Unfortunately, the data shows otherwise.

Cochrane is an independent organization that does not accept commercial or conflicted funding. They strive to provide accessible, credible information to support informed decision-making regarding healthcare. I have generally found the studies produced by Cochrane reliable over the years.

A comprehensive Cochrane review of more than 51 studies involving over 290,000 children found "…no evidence that injecting children 6-24 months of age with a flu shot was any more effective than a placebo. In children over two years, it was effective only 33% of the time in preventing the flu."[2] In other words, the flu vaccine failed 67% of children who received it.

The CDC claims high-risk individuals—patients with chronic health conditions such as asthma—are at a risk of complications from influenza. A study found that the Flumist vaccine "…did not provide any protection against hospitalizations in pediatric subjects, especially children with asthma. On the contrary, we found a [300%] increased risk of hospitalization in subjects who did get the Flumist vaccine."[3] Another study of 800 children with asthma reproted that flu vaccination failed to prevent pediatric asthma exacerbations.[4]

Is the Flu Vaccine Helpful for Adults?

So, perhaps the flu vaccine is not helpful for children, but it must be effective for adults, right? The main reason the CDC and the powers-that-be recommend flu vaccines for everyone is to prevent the complications of flu, including pneumonia, which kills over 30,000 Americans each year, especially the elderly. A Cochrane study of 52 trials of over 80,000 people looked at the safety and effectiveness of inactivated influenza vaccines in adults.[5] The authors reported that 71 healthy adults need to be vaccinated against influenza to prevent one of them experiencing influenza. In other words, 70 out of 71 (98.6%) patients received no benefit. In influenza-like illnesses, 29 healthy adults need to be vaccinated to prevent one case. This means that 28 out of 29 subjects (96.6%) received no benefit. There was no significant reduction in hospitalization among the immunized when compared to those who did not receive the flu vaccine.

A Cochrane review of 50 studies encompassing over 70,000 adults found that "...100 people need to be vaccinated to avoid one set of influenza symptoms (fever, runny nose, cough, etc.,). Vaccine use did not affect the number of people hospitalized or working days lost but caused one case of Guillain-Barré syndrome (a major neurological condition leading to paralysis) for every one million vaccinations. Our results may be an ***optimistic*** [my emphasis] estimate because company-sponsored influenza vaccine trials tend to produce results favorable to their products..."[6]

Let me review that summary. The authors state that flu vaccine does not affect the number of people hospitalized, can cause a serious neurological condition, and that even the small positive results found may be overly optimistic because Big Pharma Cartel-sponsored research results may be skewed to show only the positive results Big Pharma wants.

Flu shots for everyone? I tend to disagree.

Influenza Vaccine and the Elderly

So, the flu vaccine is virtually useless in children (and may cause harm in those children with asthma) and adults, but one would assume that it must help the elderly. In fact, the CDC and other powers-that-be scare the elderly on an annual basis, claiming that the flu vaccine is a must for people age 50 and older and people who live in nursing homes and other long-term care facilities. A Cochrane review of 75 studies found that vaccinating the elderly was ineffective at preventing the complications from the flu.[7] In fact, the researchers commented, "The available evidence supporting the use of the flu vaccine in the elderly is of such poor quality the studies provide *no guidance [emphasis added]* on the safety of the flu vaccine."

In 2018, Cochrane Database for Systemic Reviews revisited this topic and published a paper titled, "Vaccines for preventing influenza in the elderly."[8]

Cochrane reported that 30 elderly people need a flu vaccine to prevent one case of influenza and 42 would need to be vaccinated to prevent one case of influenza-like illness. That means that the flu vaccine failed to protect 29 out of 30 who received it— in other words, the flu vaccine failed 96.6% who received it. For influenza-like illnesses, it failed 41 out of 42 or 97.6%. The Cochrane authors conclude, "The evidence for a lower risk of influenza and [influenza-like illness] by vaccination is limited by biases in the design or conduct of the studies. The available evidence… provides *no clear guidance* [emphasis added] for public health regarding the safety, efficacy, or effectiveness of influenza vaccines for people aged 65 years or older."[9] And yet, influenza vaccine is recommended on an annual basis for not only all seniors, but virtually every citizen older than six months—and there is good data that the vaccine fails the vast majority who receives it.

Influenza Vaccine and Pregnant Women

The flu shot is also recommended for pregnant women even though there has never been a single study demonstrating that it is safe and effective to do so. Cochrane studied the efficacy of influenza vaccination during pregnancy versus placebo.[10] One trial involving 2,116 women was reviewed. There was no clear difference between those who received the influenza vaccine and placebo group in terms of the primary outcomes: maternal death, infant death up to 175 days after birth, perinatal death (stillbirth or death within first seven days after birth), and influenza-like illness in women or their babies or any respiratory illness in women or their babies. There was a slight reduction in polymerase-chain-reaction (PCR) confirmed influenza among infants and women. However, PCR testing for influenza is fraught with false negative tests.

Influenza vaccine has also been associated with an increased risk of miscarriages. A 2017 case-control study over two influenza seasons (2011-2012) found women who received the influenza-vaccine in two consecutive years had a six-fold higher risk of miscarriage.[11]

Influenza Vaccine and Coronavirus Infection

The powers-that-be have been stating, since the beginning of the coronavirus pandemic, that we need to continue getting the flu vaccine. However, they fail to point out that the flu vaccine has been shown to *increase* the risk for getting coronavirus as well as other influenza-like viral illnesses. This phenomenon is referred to as vaccine-associated viral interference.

Vaccine-associated viral interference is a situation where a vaccine against one illness disrupts the ability of the immune system to effectively respond to another viral illness. In other words, vaccinated individuals may be at increased risk for other respiratory viruses because they do not receive the non-specific immunity associated with a natural infection. This has been described previously in the medical literature in multiple studies relating to the influenza vaccine. One study found children immunized with the inactivated flu vaccine had a 4.4-fold increased risk of developing a virologically-confirmed non-influenza infection.[12]

A U.S. Department of Defense study investigated whether the influenza vaccine increased the risk of other respiratory viruses.[13] The author reported that flu-vaccinated individuals were found to have a 36% increase risk of coronavirus when compared to those not vaccinated. There continue to be more studies showing the flu vaccine increases the risk of other viral illnesses. These studies include:

- A 2018 CDC study found flu shots were associated with a 65% increase risk of respiratory illnesses including coronavirus in children.[14]
- A 2017 Jackson, MS study found a 490% increase risk in pneumonia in vaccinated versus unvaccinated children.[15]

Final Thoughts

When the final statistics for the COVID-19 pandemic are released, it will be interesting to see if those vaccinated with the influenza vaccine show either an increased, decreased, or no change in infection susceptibility to SARS-CoV-2, the virus that causes COVID-19. In other words, did the flu vaccine make people more or less susceptible to coronavirus infection? Recall the earlier study I wrote about, which found a 36% increase risk in coronavirus infection in those that received the influenza vaccine.[16]

My patients are asking me what to do about the coronavirus vaccine. Should they take it or not? My current advice is to wait and see. I hope the coronavirus vaccine is both safe and effective. As for the safety profile, keep in mind this is a "warp-speed" project. Many safety steps are being omitted. As for the efficacy of the new vaccines, time will tell. The advice I have given to my patients is this: I would not be first in line for any "warp-speed" produced vaccine.

[1] https://www.cdc.gov/mmwr/volumes/67/rr/rr6703a1.htm?s_cid=rr6703a1_w
[2] Vaccines for preventing influenza in healthy children." The Cochrane Database of Systematic Reviews. 2 (2008).
[3] The American Thoracic Society's 105th International Conference, May 15-20, 2009, San Diego. C94 VIRAL INFECTIONS IN CHILDHOOD RESPIRATORY DISEASE / Mini Symposium / Tuesday, May 19/1:30 PM–4:00 PM
[4] Arch Dis Child. 2004 Aug;89(8):734-5.
[5] Demicheli V, Jefferson T, Ferroni E, Rivetti A, Di Pietrantonj C. Vaccines for preventing influenza in healthy adults. Cochrane Database of Systematic Reviews 2018, Issue 2. Art. No.: CD001269. DOI: 10.1002/14651858.CD001269.pub6.
[6] Vaccines for preventing influenza in healthy adults (Review) 115
Copyright © 2010 The Cochrane Collaboration
[7] Cochrane Database of Systematic Reviews 2010, Issue 2. Art. No.: CD004876. DOI: 10.1002/14651858.CD004876.pub3
[8] Demicheli V, Jefferson T, Di Pietrantonj C, Ferroni E, Thorning S, Thomas RE, Rivetti A. Vaccines for preventing influenza in the elderly. Cochrane Database of Systematic Reviews 2018, Issue 2. Art. No.: CD004876. DOI: 10.1002/14651858.CD004876.pub4
[9] Demicheli, V., et al. IBID. 2018.
[10] Salam RA, Das JK, Dojo Soeandy C, Lassi ZS, Bhutta ZA. Impact of *Haemophilus influenzae* type B (Hib) and viral influenza vaccinations in pregnancy for improving maternal, neonatal and infant health outcomes. Cochrane Database of Systematic Reviews 2015, Issue 6. Art. No.: CD009982. DOI: 10.1002/14651858.CD009982.pub2.
[11] Donahue JG, Kieke BA, King JP, et al. Association of spontaneous abortion with receipt of inactivated influenza vaccine containing H1N1pdm09 in 2010-11 and 2011-12. *Vaccine*. 2017;35(40):5314-5322. doi:10.1016/j.vaccine.2017.06.069.
[12] Benjamin J. Cowling, Vicky J. Fang, Hiroshi Nishiura, Kwok-Hung Chan, Sophia Ng, Dennis K. M. Ip, Susan S. Chiu, Gabriel M. Leung, J. S. Malik Peiris, Increased Risk of Noninfluenza Respiratory Virus Infections Associated With Receipt of Inactivated Influenza Vaccine, *Clinical Infectious Diseases*, Volume 54, Issue 12, 15 June 2012, Pages 1778–1783, https://doi.org/10.1093/cid/cis307
[13] Wolff, Greg. Influenza vaccination and respiratory virus interference among Department of Defense personnel during the 2017–2018 influenza season. Vaccine. Vol. 38;2: January 10, 2020.p.350-354.
[14] Rikin, Sharon, et al. Assessment of temporally-related acute respiratory illness following influenza vaccination. Vaccine. 36; 2018. 1958-1964
[15] Mawson, Anthony R, et al. Pilot comparative study on the health of vaccinated and unvaccinated 6- to 12-year-old U.S. children. J Transl Sci, Vol. 3(3). 2017p. 1-12. doi: 10.15761/JTS.1000186
[16] Wolff, Gregg. IBID. January 10, 2020.

Chapter 12

This Is Our Wakeup Call

This is Our Wake-Up Call

As of this writing we are still suffering the ravages of SARS-CoV-2. The Centers for Disease Control and Prevention (CDC) report that in the US, there are 7,824,485 total cases of SARS-CoV-2, the virus that causes COVID-19. We have suffered 217,485 deaths from coronavirus. And, we are not done with it yet. Over the last seven days, the CDC reports 335,009 new cases of COVID-19.[1]

Keep in mind, these numbers are being reported even though we had a near total lockdown for months and we are wearing masks and social distancing. Many businesses are still closed and, unfortunately, far too many will never reopen. The economic devastation from COVID-19 is beyond words.

The fear is palpable everywhere. People are arguing in stores about mask wearing. I have heard strangers confronting one another, shaming and name calling, because they feel others are not taking this pandemic seriously enough. Walking my dog (Patch the Wonder Dog) on a path in the woods, I pass by strangers who are wearing masks outside while walking, riding a bike or jogging. Some even turn their backs to me and flee because I do not wear a mask when outside.

In regard to COVID-19, two questions come to mind: How did we get to this place? How will we get over this?

The answer to these questions is crucial. We need to get out of this mess and prevent a similar situation from occurring in the future.

How Did We Get to This Place?

COVID-19 should not be a surprise to anyone. The only thing I am surprised about is that it took so long for something like this to happen to us. And, keep in mind, after COVID-19 there will be other viruses to contend with.

I have been writing, lecturing, and studying holistic medicine for over 25 years. During this time, I have seen a gradual and steady decline in the health of Americans. We finish last or next to last on *every health indicator* when compared with other Western countries. Simply put, we are an unhealthy society.

My medical training taught me very little about health. In fact, I am being generous by saying "very little" here. As I previously stated, I was trained in a disease model where I learned to diagnose pathologies and prescribe drugs to treat the diagnoses. The drugs I was well trained to use did not promote health. In fact, they did the opposite. Well over 95% of prescription drugs (my estimate) work by poisoning enzymes and blocking receptors in the human body. There is a time and a place to use drugs like that, such as during an acute situation like a heart attack. However, the long-term use of these drugs does the opposite of promoting health: they block and poison physiology and biochemistry.

Americans take more prescription medicines than any people on the planet. We spend nearly twenty percent of our GDP on health care. And the results are disastrous.

Why do we take so many prescription medications? We take these drugs because we are an unhealthy society, and doctors have little knowledge about how to promote health.

COVID-19 hit Americans so hard because we were a very unhealthy society going into the illness. Two-thirds of Americans are overweight, and one-third are obese. We have obese children now. When I was a child, an obese child was not a common sight—it was a rare thing. In 2011, scientists reported that over 50% of our children suffer from a chronic illness.[2] The same article reports that

21% of US children are developmentally disabled. That was in 2011. Things are worse now.

Folks, these numbers are tragic. Why aren't the powers-that-be talking about this? As I write this book, the presidential election is in full swing. Neither party speaks the truth about what is going on with our health. Instead, they praise themselves for doing little, while more and more die of treatable and/or preventable illnesses including COVID-19.

But, all is not bleak. We can change the trajectory of where we are going.

How Will We Get Over This?

The answer to the above question is easy: Adopt a holistic lifestyle. It may not be easy to start this program, and will take a lot of work, but it can be done. And, it will be worth it.

Daily, I see patients who have gone down the wrong path in relation to their health. Once we partner together, we can design a plan to alter this path and improve their health. My job is to identify where the physiology and biochemistry are not being properly supported and explain it to the patient. Then we work together to rectify the situation such as correcting nutritional and hormonal imbalances. In addition, detoxifying heavy metals and other toxins aids the physiology. Eating a healthy diet and drinking water helps every situation. Identifying and avoiding or treating food allergies can lower inflammatory levels. And, I cannot emphasize enough the power of exercise.

When my patients adopt a holistic plan, oftentimes they can stop taking medications for chronic conditions including diabetes, hypertension, heart disease, asthma, arthritis, and autoimmune illnesses. That is why I write my books, blogs, and newsletters. It makes the practice of medicine worthwhile when I observe patients making changes in their daily routines that support their physiology and biochemistry so that their health improves and their illnesses go away. This is the core reason why I went into medicine.

COVID-19 Is Our Wake-up Call

It deserves repeating: *COVID-19 is our wake-up call*. We can do better. We must do better, or we will not leave a country that is viable for our children or our grandchildren. We are at a crossroads: It is time for each and every one of us to take responsibility for our own health decisions. We must learn about how and why we should eat healthy foods. We must be able to identify unhealthy foods and avoid them. We all need to learn about how best to support and nourish a healthy immune system.

You cannot depend on anyone else but yourself to do this. Education is the key. When you are ready, I have a few (16!) books for you to read! I have seen holistic medicine work for me, my family, and my patients. I see and hear about the positive results daily.

We do not have to suffer poor health. We should not stand for it and we were not designed for it.

COVID-19 is indeed our wake-up call. So, let's **WAKE UP,** shake off the cobwebs, and adopt healthier ways. If you don't have a holistic doctor, it is past time to find one. *

To All Our Health,

DrB

*I recommend finding a holistic doctor at the International College of Integrative Medicine (www.icimed.com) where I currently am a member and on the board of directors.

[1] Accessed 10.11.20 from: https://covid.cdc.gov/covid-data-tracker/#cases_casesinlast7days

[2] Bethell, Christina, et al. A National and State Profile of Leading Health Problems and Health Care Quality for US Children: Key Insurance Disparities and Across-State Variations. Academic Pediatrics. Vol. 11:3 supplement: May-June 2011, p. S22-S33.

Appendix

Appendix

Science, Public Health Policy, and The Law
Volume 2:4-22
July, 2020
Clinical and Translational Research

An Institute for Pure
and Applied Knowledge (IPAK)
Public Health Policy
Initiative (PHPI)

IPAK PHPI

A Novel Approach to Treating COVID-19 Using Nutritional and Oxidative Therapies

David Brownstein, M.D. *†, Richard Ng, M.D. †, Robert Rowen, M.D. ‡, Jennie-Dare Drummond , PA †, Taylor Eason, NP †, Hailey Brownstein, D.O. §, and Jessica Brownstein ¶

Abstract

Objective: This report is a case series of consecutive patients diagnosed with **COVID-19** treated with a nutritional and oxidative medical approach. We describe the treatment program and report the response of the 107 **COVID-19** patients.

Study Design: Observational case series consecutive.

Setting: A family practice office in a suburb of Detroit, Michigan.

Patients: All patients seen in the office from February through May 2020 diagnosed with **COVID-19** were included in the study. **COVID-19** was either diagnosed via PCR or antibody testing as well as those not tested diagnosed via symptomology.

Interventions: Oral Vitamins A, C, D, and iodine were given to 107 subjects (99%). Intravenous solutions of hydrogen peroxide and Vitamin C were given to 32 (30%) and 37 (35%) subjects. Thirty-seven (35%) of the cohort was treated with intramuscular ozone. A dilute, nebulized hydrogen peroxide/saline mixture, with Lugol's iodine, was used by 91 (85%).

Main Outcome Measures: History and physical exam were reviewed for **COVID-19** symptoms including cough, fever, shortness of breath, and gastrointestinal complaints. Laboratory reports were examined for **SARS-CoV-2** results. Symptomatic improvement after treatment was reported for each patient consisting of *first improvement, mostly better,* and *completely better.*

continued on next page

Keywords
SARS-CoV-2, COVID-19, ozone therapy, hydrogen peroxide therapy, Vitamin A, iodine, Vitamin C, Vitamin D, immune system, antiviral.

---

*Clinical Assistant Professor of Family Medicine, Wayne State University School of Medicine. Corresponding author, **info@drbrownstein.com**

†private practice West Bloomfield, MI

‡private practice Santa Rosa, CA.

§resident physician, Providence Hospital, Southfield, MI

¶4th year Michigan State College of Osteopathic Medicine student

Contents

Abstract (Continued from page 1)
Results: There were a total of 107 patients diagnosed with **COVID-19**. Thirty-four were tested for SARS-CoV-2(32%) and twenty-seven (25%) tested positive. Three were hospitalized (3%) with two of the three hospitalized before instituting treatment and only one requiring hospitalization after beginning treatment. There were no deaths. The most common symptoms in the cohort were fever (81%), shortness of breath (68%), URI which included cough (69%), and gastrointestinal distress symptoms (27%). For the entire cohort, first improvement was noted in 2.4 days. The cohort reported symptoms mostly better after 4.4 days and completely better 6.9 days after starting the program. For the **SARS-CoV-2** test positive patients, fever was present in 25 (93%), shortness of breath in 20 (74%) and upper respiratory symptoms including cough in 21 (78%) while gastrointestinal symptoms were present in 9 (33%). The time to improvement in the **SARS-CoV-2** test positive group was slightly longer than the entire cohort.
Conclusion: At present, there is no published cure, treatment, or preventive for **COVID-19** except for a recent report on dexamethasone for seriously ill patients. A novel treatment program combining nutritional and oxidative therapies was shown to successfully treat the signs and symptoms of 100% of 107 patients diagnosed with **COVID-19**. Each patient was treated with an individualized plan consisting of a combination of oral, IV, IM, and nebulized nutritional and oxidative therapies which resulted in zero deaths and recovery from **COVID-19**. Keywords: **SARS-CoV-2**, COVID-19, ozonc therapy, hydrogen peroxie therapy, Vitamin A, iodine, Vitamin C, Vitamin D, immune system, antiviral.

1. Introduction

SARS-CoV-2 is the strain of coronavirus that causes coronavirus disease 2019 known as **COVID-19**. To date, **COVID-19** has infected 7,669,872 cases worldwide and 2,090,553 cases in the US with 116,347 reported fatalities (as of 6.13.2020).[1] **COVID-19** is a pandemic that is unparalleled in the modern world and the global response to **SARS-CoV-2** has no parallel in history. Coronaviruses are found in many bat and bird species, which are believed to be natural hosts.[2] It is estimated that coronaviruses have been around from 10,000 to millions of years. Coronaviruses are pathogenic viruses native to birds and mammals. They are classified into four subspecies: alpha-, beta-, gamma-, and delta- coronavirus.[3] Alpha- and beta- coronaviruses are found exclusively in mammals and gamma- and delta-coronavirus primarily infect birds.[4] Coronaviruses include a family of viruses that contain an RNA genome. Some of these viruses have been shown to cause illness in animals and humans.

SARS (severe acute respiratory syndrome) was discovered in 2003.[5] It was described as an outbreak of atypical pneumonia in Guangdong Province, Peoples Republic of China. SARS, which occurred during 2002-2003 infected approximately 8,098 and resulted in 774 deaths. The outbreak was primarily concentrated in Southeast Asia and Toronto, Canada although the outbreak spread to more than 24 countries. SARS was found to be caused by a strain of coronavirus that infects the epithelial lining within the lungs.[6] Prior to the SARS outbreak, coronaviruses were only thought to cause mild influenza-like illnesses in humans.

The second major human outbreak of coronavirus was in 2012 in Saudi Arabia. It was referred to as MERS (Middle East Respiratory Syndrome). It spread to several countries including the US. Most people infected with MERS suffered with respiratory problems including cough and shortness of breath. The World Health Organization confirmed 2,519 cases of MERS as of January, 2020.[7]

SARS-CoV-2 is a new strain of coronavirus that has not been known to previously infect humans.

COVID-19 was first identified in Wuhan, China in December 2019. China informed the WHO that a novel strain of coronavirus was causing severe illness. It was named **SARS-CoV-2** as the cause of **COVID-19**. The virus was sequenced and found to most resemble viruses found in bats and pangolins.[8] **SARS-CoV-2** was found to be highly transmissible between humans. **SARS-CoV-2** can be diagnosed via nasal swab PCR testing. According the Centers for Disease Control and Prevention, people with **COVID-19** have a wide range of symptoms reported from mild symptoms to severe illness.[9] People with these symptoms may have **COVID-19**:

- Cough

- Shortness of Breath or difficulty breathing

Or at least two of these symptoms:

- Fever

- Chills

- Repeated shaking with chills

- Muscle pain

- Headache

- Sore throat

- New loss of taste or smell

The CDC further states, that this list is not inclusive. According the CDC, the signs and symptoms of **COVID-19** present at illness vary, but over the course of the disease, most persons with **COVID-19** will experience the following:[10]

- Fever (83-99%)

- Cough (59-82%)

- Shortness of breath (31-40%)

- Sputum production (28-33%)

Our patients' symptomology correlated well with the percentages reported by the CDC.

We will present data on clinical presentation and treatment provided to help patients recover from **COVID-19** symptoms. This treatment program has been utilized for over 20 years (with some variations) in treating patients suffering from viral illnesses such as influenza-like disease. This treatment program was not designed to cure a viral illness rather its purpose is to provide a therapeutic regimen designed to support the immune system when it is challenged with a viral infection.

2. Methods

The setting for this retrospective review is an outpatient medical office (referred to as CHM) consisting of five practitioners. The office is in the metropolitan Detroit area, which was one of the hot spots for **COVID-19**. The practitioners include three medical doctors as well as a nurse practitioner and a physician's assistant. For the calendar year of 2020, charts were retrospectively reviewed for the presence of **COVID-19** diagnosis occurring from February 2020 through May 2020. The charts were analyzed for clinical symptoms, physical findings, imaging and coronavirus testing results. Additionally, the charts were analyzed for interventions provided and duration to relief of symptoms. Three endpoints were taken from the charts – hospitalization, death, and time to improvement.

All patients gave fully informed consent for integrative medical management of their condition. Historical information from the charts included age, sex, birthdate, initial date of service, care provider, past medical history, medications, and nutritional supplements. The number of days of illness prior to being seen by a provider was documented as well.

For x-ray imaging we used the report provided by the radiologist. Coronavirus testing was done through outpatient and inpatient laboratories. Coronavirus was diagnosed by PCR nasal swab testing.

The interventions provided at the outpatient medical office included oral supplementation of iodine, Vitamins A, C and D, intravenous hydrogen peroxide and Vitamin C, intramuscular ozone injections, and a nebulized solution of dilute hydrogen peroxide and iodine.

Oral dosing consisted of taking the following supplements for four days at the first sign of symptoms or at the direction of the practitioner. The supplements consisted of:

- Vitamin A: 100,000 IU/day*** in the form of emulsified Vitamin A palmitate

- Vitamin C: 1,000 mg/hour while awake in the form of ascorbic acid until bowel tolerance (loose stools) was reached

- Vitamin D3: 50,000 IU/day in an emulsified form

- Iodine: 25 mg/day in the form of Lugol's solution or tableted Lugol's solution

Most patients were instructed to nebulize a dilute solution of 0.04% hydrogen peroxide in normal saline. The solution was mixed for the patient in the office. A sterile 250 cc bag of normal saline was injected with 3 cc of 3% food grade hydrogen peroxide and 1 cc of magnesium sulfate. The patient was instructed to draw off 3 cc of the dilute solution and nebulize it hourly until symptoms improve. Additionally, the patient was instructed to add in one drop of 5% Lugol's solution to the dilute hydrogen peroxide mixture. As the symptoms improved, the frequency of nebulizing could be reduced by the patient.

If symptoms worsened or there was a concern that the patient was suffering from a more severe case, the patient was advised to come to the office and receive intravenous injections of Vitamin C and hydrogen peroxide along with intramuscular injections of ozone. The dosing of these items is shown below:

- Vitamin C: 2.5 grams of sodium ascorbate (5 cc of a 500 mg/cc ascorbic acid solution) mixed with an equal amount of sterile water given as an intravenous push over 2-3 minutes.

Age in years

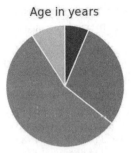

■ 0-25 ■ 26-50 ■ 51-75 ■ 76+
Figure 1. Patient Age distribution

- Hydrogen peroxide: 30 cc of a 0.03% solution of dilute hydrogen peroxide given as an intravenous push over 2-3 minutes

- Ozone: 20 cc of 18 mcg/cc ozone (as an oxygen/ozone gas mixture) given in each buttock as an intramuscular injection

3. Results

There were 107 patients identified in our chart review among five practitioners. **Table I** outlines the patient characteristics of the sample. The age of patients ranges from 2-85 years old with an average age of 54.2 and median age of 56.5. 80 patients were female (75%) and 27 were male (25%). The major comorbid conditions of the sample include hypothyroidism (18%), hypertension (10%), asthma (8%), Lyme disease (6%), Hashimoto's disease (5%), cigarette smoking (3%), Grave's disease (2%), chronic sinusitis (2%), diabetes (2%) and cancer (2%).

Figure 1 exemplifies the age distribution of the 107-patient population at the practice. The majority of the patients were between 51-75 years old (59%). The second highest cohort was between 26-50 years old (31%). Followed by those 76 years old and older (10%) and those aged 2-25 (7%).

Table II illustrates the patient symptoms of the total cohort. The most common patient symptom was fever (81%), shortness of breath (68%), URI (69%) and GI symptoms (27%).

Table 1. Patient Characteristics

	N(%)
Total patients	107(100)
Age	
Range	2-85
Average	54.2
Median	56.5
Sex	
Male	27 (25)
Female	80 (75)
Comorbid Conditions	
Hypothyroidism	19 (18)
Hypertension	11 (10)
Asthma	9 (8)
Lyme Disease	6 (6)
Hashimoto's disease	5 (5)
Smokers	3 (3)
Grave's disease	2 (2)
Chronic sinusitis	2 (2)
Diabetes	2 (2)
Cancer	2 (2)

Table 2. Patient Symptoms 'Total Cohort'

	N (%)
Fever	87 (81)
Shortness of breath	73 (68)
URI (symptoms including cough)	74 (69)
GI (diarrhea, loose stools, pain)	29 (27)
Total patients	107 (100)**

Table 3 demonstrates the interventions that the patients received from CHM (total cohort). The most common intervention was a protocol of oral supplements, including Vitamin A, Vitamin D, Vitamin C, and iodine. 106 patients of the 107 total patients were taking oral supplements (99%). The other interventions at CHM include 32 patients receiving IV hydrogen peroxide (30%), 37 patients receiving IV Vitamin C (35%), 37 patients receiving intramuscular ozone injections (35%), 91 patients receiving a nebulized solution of normal saline and dilute hydrogen peroxide (85%), and 91 patients receiving nebulized iodine (85%).

Figure 2 shows the average number of days that patient reported symptomatic improvement after CHM interventions (for total cohort). On average, patients reported their first improvement by 2.4 days following CHM interventions. Patients reported feeling mostly better by 4.4 days following interventions. Patients reported feeling completely better after 6.9 days following CHM interventions.

Table 4 illustrates the disease course in the total cohort. 34 of the 107 total patients (32%) were tested for COVID-19. Of those 34 tested, 27 patients tested positive for COVID-19 (79%). Therefore, 25% of the entire cohort (107 patients) had tested positive for COVID-19.[1] Of the total 107 patients, 0 died (0%).

Table 5 illustrates the symptoms of the COVID-19 cohort which was similar to **Table 2** for the entire cohort.[2] **Figure 3** shows the symptomatic improvement after intervention in the **SARS-CoV-2** laboratory positive cohort. Compared to the entire cohort (**Figure 2**), there was approximately a one day longer time period to feeling *mostly better* and *completely better* for those who tested positive for **SARS-CoV-2** as reported by the patients.

---

[1]Of the 107 total patients, three were hospitalized (3%) with two of the three hospitalized before beginning treatment.

[2]Two patients in the SARS-CoV-2 positive cohort reported a return of mild symptoms after reporting a resolution of major symptoms. One patient reported feeling foggy in his head and another reported a fast heart (90-100 bpm) along with mild shortness of breath with any mild exertional activity. A workup onboth failed to find a cause for the symptoms.

Table 3. Patient Interventions

INTERVENTION	total (cohort) N (%)
Total patients	107 (100)**
Oral supplements	106 (99)
IV H2O2	32 (30)
IV Vitamin C	37 (35)
IM Ozone	37 (35)
Nebulized NS/H2O2	91 (85)
Nebulized Iodine	91 (85)

Table 4. Disease Course

	N (%)
Total cohort	107 (100)
Tested for COVID-19	34 (32)
Tested positive for COVID-19	27 (25)
Hospitalized	3 (3) *
Death	0 (0)

* Of the three patients hospitalized, two were hospitalized before instituting treatment. One was hospitalized on the oral Vitamin regimen of Vitamins A, C, D, and iodine. All three made a full recovery and were treated with nebulized hydrogen peroxide and iodine.

Table 5. Symptoms of COVID-19 Positive Cohort

	N (%)
COVID positive patients	27 (100)**
Fever	25 (93)
Shortness of breath	20 (74)
URI (includes cough)	21 (78)
GI	9 (33)

**Two patients in the SARS-CoV-2 positive cohort reported a return of mild symptoms after reporting a resolution of major symptoms. One patient reported feeling foggy in his head and another reported a fast heart (90-100 bpm) along with mild shortness of breath with any mild exertional activity. A workup on both failed to find a cause for the symptoms.

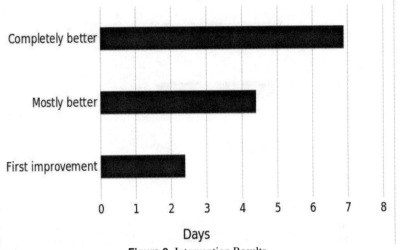

Figure 2. Intervention Results

4. Discussion

COVID-19 is a worldwide pandemic caused by coronavirus. Currently, there is no vaccine or cure for **COVID-19**. Dexamethasone has been reported to reduce hospitalized case mortality.[11] Those who have recovered from **COVID-19** have done so because their immune system was successful in fighting off the illness. Therefore, a successful treatment for **COVID-19** will have to either have viricidal activity or work by aiding the immune system's response in fighting the pathogen. Many feel **COVID-19** will come back during the next flu season—fall/winter of 2020-2021. Therefore, there is an urgent need for any therapy that supports the host's immune system and allows for an uneventful recovery from the illness.

This cohort study consisted of a retrospective review of 107 patients who were either diagnosed as **COVID-19** positive by PCR nasal swab testing or presumed to have **COVID-19** due to symptomatology. The most common symptom in our cohort was fever. The fever was reported as fluctuating varying between 99-102 degrees Fahrenheit for most sub-

jects. The next most common symptom included upper respiratory symptoms which included a rhinorrhea, drippy eyes, cough, and congestion. Shortness of breath was the third most common complaint. Gastrointestinal distress, though common, was lower on the symptom list. Although symptoms varied between patients, all patients exhibited symptoms that could be consistent with a viral pathology.

Treatments of the cohort consisted of first using oral nutrient therapies. The vast majority—91 (88%) started taking vitamins A, C, D3 and iodine at the first sign of a viral illness such as a cough, runny nose, sore throat, etc., All subjects (100%) took vitamin C in suggested doses of at least 3-5,000 mg/day of ascorbic acid. Three patients took vitamins C and D only.

There were three hospitalizations in the cohort group. One patient was taking the oral protocol of vitamins A, C, D and iodine when he became ill with a cough and fever. His condition worsened over the next seven days and was admitted to the hospital where he was diagnosed with pneumonia. He was treated with antibiotics. He phoned the

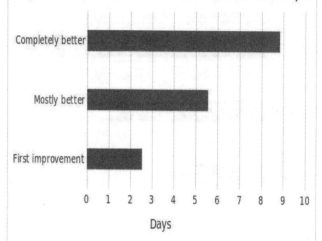

Figure 3. *Two patients in the **SARS-CoV-2** positive cohort reported a return of mild symptoms after reporting a resolution of major symptoms. One patient reported feeling foggy in his head and another reported a fast heart (90-100 bpm) along with mild shortness of breath with any mild exertional activity. A workup on both failed to find a cause for the symptoms.

office after he was discharged from the hospital because he was having breathing difficulties. He started nebulizing hydrogen peroxide and felt an immediate improvement in his breathing difficulties from this therapy. By the third nebulized therapy he reported to being 80% improved. He stated his breathing difficulties began to return to normal after day two of nebulizing every 2 hours while awake. The other two patients started our protocol after

being hospitalized for **COVID-19**. One of the two was recently diagnosed with acute myelogenous leukemia and recently received chemotherapy. Both were discharged still symptomatic with breathing difficulties and a severe cough. Both patients were treated with nebulized hydrogen peroxide and iodine as well as the oral protocol of vitamins A, C, D, and iodine. All three patients fully recovered.

4.1 Vitamin A

Vitamin A consists of a group of retinoid compounds that have a wide range of physiological effects including the support of immune system functioning. Vitamin A deficiency is a worldwide problem affecting 250 million preschool children and half of all countries.[12] In children, vitamin A supplementation has been shown to dramatically decrease the mortality from the viral illnesses such as measles and diarrheal infections.[13]

Over 100 years ago, — before the chemical structure was elucidated — studies of vitamin A pointed to its important role in immune system functioning. Fat in butter, a good source of vitamin A, improved the outcome of infections in malnourished animals and humans.[14] Rats were shown to be more susceptible to infections when they were vitamin A deficient.[15] Vitamin A is fundamental in maintaining the integrity of the epithelium.[16] Vitamin A deficiency has been associated with disruptions in normal epithelium of the respiratory tract[17][18] and gastrointestinal tissue.[19][20] Vitamin A has been shown to be an important regulator of monocyte differentiation and function.[21]

COVID-19 is characterized by cytokine storm in the severely ill.[22] Therapies that lower cytokine formation are being investigated. Retinoic acid, when added to monocytic, myelomonocytic, or dendritic cell line cultures promotes cellular differentiation and influences the secretion of key cytokines produced by macrophages including TNF-α, IL-1β, Il-6, and IL-12. It has been hypothesized that supplementation with preformed vitamin A may down-regulate the secretion of specific proinflammatory cytokines such as TNF- α and Il-6 by macrophages.[23]

Acute respiratory distress syndrome (ARDS) accompanied by respiratory failure is a major cause of death from **COVID-19**.[24][25] Treatments to combat respiratory failure are urgently needed.

In vitro and *in vivo* studies have found that IgA antibodies can neutralize intracellular pathogens including viruses by inhibiting or blocking their attachment to epithelial cells.[26][27][28] Researchers studying the acute humoral response to **SARS-CoV-2** in serum and bronchoalveolar fluid of 145 patients with **COVID-19** reported that early **SARS-CoV-2** specific humoral responses were found to be typically dominated by antibodies of the IgA isotype.[29] Furthermore, the subjects who had the highest levels of IgA against the spike protein for **SARS-CoV-2** were the ones who had the greatest ability to neutralize the virus. Vitamin A deficiency has been shown to inhibit the production of influenza-specific IgA in mice.[30] Furthermore, vitamin A supplementation has been shown to increase IgA levels.[31]

4.2 Vitamin C (Ascorbate)

A Chinese report of intravenous vitamin C (IVC) infusion for 50 moderate to severe **COVID-19** subjects found all patients eventually recovered and discharged from the hospital. The subjects were given between 10 and 20 g of IVC per day over a period of 8-10 hours.[32] In 2017, Paul Marik, M.D. developed a protocol for treating septic patients

with IV vitamin C, thiamine, and hydrocortisone. The early use of vitamin C along with thiamine and hydrocortisone were found to be effective at preventing progressive organ dysfunction including kidney injury and in reducing mortality of patients with severe sepsis and septic shock. In CITRIS-ALI researchers reported a trial where ARDS patients were randomized to receive IV ascorbic acid or placebo every six hours for 4 days. Patients had to develop ARDS within 24 hours of ICU admission. The authors reported a reduction in 28-day all-cause mortality rate in those receiving IV vitamin C: 29.8% mortality in the treatment group versus 46.3% mortality in the placebo group.[33] **COVID-19** patients are characterized by elevated levels of inflammatory markers and oxidative stress such as hsCRP.[34] Vitamin C is known to have anti-oxidant and anti-inflammatory effects. Erythrocytes (red blood cells) can deliver oxygen to bodily tissues because they carry iron-containing hemoglobin which reversibly binds oxygen. Oxidative damage to red blood cells can impair the ability to deliver oxygen to tissues.[35] The management (and possibly the prevention of) oxidative stress in **COVID-19** may be addressed with the use of anti-oxidant therapies. High-dose IV vitamin C was found to have an antioxidant effect for lung epithelial cells.[36] Vitamin C has also been shown to prevent the oxidation of iron from its reduced ferrous state to the oxidized ferric form.[37] Intravenous (but not oral) ascorbate has been shown to act as a pro-drug for hydrogen peroxide creation in interstitial fluids in animal studies (see hydrogen peroxide discussion below).[38]

4.3 Vitamin D

Vitamin D is being researched as an effective treatment option for **COVID-19** patients. Researchers used 25-hydroxyVitamin D [25(OH)D] levels as a marker to predict clinical outcomes of **COVID-19** subjects.[39] Of 212 cases of **COVID-19**, serum 25(OH)D level was lowest in critical cases but highest in mild cases. The authors reported vitamin D is significantly associated with clinical outcomes. A logistic regression analysis reported that for each standard deviation increase in serum 25(OH)D, the odds of having a mild clinical outcome rather than a severe outcome were approximately 7.94 times (OR=0.126, p<0.001) while interestingly, the odds of having a mild clinical outcome rather than a critical outcome were approximately 19.61 times (OR=0.051, p<0.001). The results suggest that an increase in serum 25(OH)D level in the body could either improve clinical outcomes or mitigate worst (severe to critical) outcomes, while a decrease in serum **25(OH)D** level in the body could worsen clinical outcomes of **COVID-2019** patients.

There are several mechanisms by which vitamin D could reduce the risk of influenza-like infections and death. Viral infections have been shown to disrupt airway epithelial cell junctions.[40] Vitamin D has been shown to maintain tight epithelial junctions and adherens junctions.[41]

Vitamin D has been shown to modulate cellular immunity and reduce cytokine storm by reducing the production of proinflammatory cytokines including TNF-α and interferon-γ as well as increasing the anti-inflammatory cytokines produced by macrophages.[42] A study comparing deceased rates for patients with **COVID-19** from countries with a large number of confirmed patients (including Germany, S. Korea, China, Switzerland, Iran, UK, US, France, Spain, and Italy) found a risk of severe **COVID-19** cases among patients with very low vitamin D levels is 17.3%, while the equivalent figure for patients with normal vitamin D levels is 14.6%–a reduction of 15.6%.

The authors hypothesized that vitamin D may reduce symptoms of **COVID-19** by suppressing cytokine storm in **COVID-19** patients.[43]

Vitamin D is produced in the bone, skin, lungs, colon, parathyroid glands, and immune system cells. Activation of vitamin D in response to viral infection has been described.[44] A deficiency of vitamin D could impair this response in the lung.[45]

4.4 Iodine

Iodine is an essential element; therefore it must be obtained from the diet or via supplementation. For over 40 years, US iodine levels have fallen in the National Health and Nutrition Examination Survey (NHANES).[46] Nearly 60% of women of childbearing age are deficient in iodine.[47] In fact, the mean urinary iodine concentration among pregnant US women is 134 ug/L which signifies deficiency.[48] We have tested over 6,000 patients and found the vast majority—over 97%– are deficient in iodine.

Iodine is needed for proper immune system functioning. Iodine supplementation has been shown to increased IgG synthesis in human lymphocytes.[49] Iodine deficiency is associated with decreased phagocytic activity of blood neutrophils.[50] This was associated with a decrease in peroxidases in neutrophils. Iodine has been shown to increase the ability of granulocytes to kill infectious organisms.[51] Iodine is used as an antiseptic throughout the US because it has antiviral and antibacterial properties. Two of us (DB and RN) have used iodine successfully as an antimicrobial agent for over two decades.

In order to reduce transmission of viruses, antisepsis of human and non-human surfaces must be identified. Researchers reported an *in-vitro* study where **SARS-2-CoV** was exposed to iodine (povidone-iodine) at 1-5% concentrations as a nasal antiseptic formulation and an oral rinse. The iodine solutions effectively inactivated **SARS-CoV-2** after exposure times of 60 seconds.[52] *In vitro* studies of 0.23% PVP-I mouthwash (1:30 dilution) was shown to inactivate both **SARS-CoV** and **MERS-CoV** following a 15-second exposure.[53]

Japan has one of the lowest rates of **COVID-19** illnesses in the Western world even in a crowded city such as Tokyo. Furthermore, Japan has not gone on a total lockdown. The Japanese are known to have a much higher iodine intake through their diet when compared to other Western countries. It is estimated that the Mainland Japanese ingest over 100x the RDA as compared to US citizens.[54] Perhaps Tokyo and Japan itself has had less serious **COVID-19** illness because of their iodine intake.

The full oral supplementation regimen (vitamins A, C, D, and iodine) in COVID-19 subjects was used in 91 out of 104 subjects in the cohort. The subjects were instructed to take the supplements for four days. Some were treated with vitamin C (1), vitamins C and D (2) and vitamins C, D, and iodine (1). All of these patients recovered without sequalae.

4.5 Nebulized Hydrogen Peroxide

If there were more serious problems or the oral supplementation regimen failed to fully help alleviate the symptoms of **COVID-19**, the next step was to initiate the use of a combination of nebulized hydrogen peroxide and iodine. A solution of 250 cc of normal saline was mixed with 3 cc of 3% hydrogen peroxide providing a final concentration of 0.04% hydrogen peroxide. (Note, the hydrogen peroxide used was initially a 35% food grade source then diluted to 3% using a 10:1 mixture of sterile water to 35% hydrogen peroxide.) Additionally, 1 cc of magnesium chloride (200 mg/ml) was added to the 250 cc saline/hydrogen peroxide bag. (This was mixed in the office for the patients.)

Patients were instructed to nebulize 3 cc of the mixture three times per day or more often if there were breathing problems. Usually one or two nebulizer treatments were reported to improve breathing problems.

A total of 91 **COVID-19** subjects (85%) utilized the nebulized solution. They reported no adverse effects. One We have been using nebulized saline/hydrogen peroxide at this concentration for over two decades in his practice.

Hydrogen peroxide is continually produced in the human body with substantial amounts produced in the mitochondria.[55] Every cell in the body is exposed to some level of hydrogen peroxide.[56] The lungs are known to produce hydrogen peroxide.[57] Nebulized hydrogen peroxide has been shown to have antiviral activities.[58] Hydrogen peroxide can activate lymphocytes[59] which are known to be depleted in **COVID-19**.

4.6 Intravenous and Intramuscular Therapies

If **COVID-19** patients continued to have symptoms such as shortness of breath, fever, or cough, they were offered intravenous injections of hydrogen peroxide, Vitamin C and intramuscular injections of ozone.

4.7 IV Hydrogen Peroxide

A dilute IV solution of hydrogen peroxide was given in either an IV drip over 30 minutes or a rapid infusion as an IV push over 2-3 minutes. One of the earliest known uses of hydrogen peroxide was used by Dr. T.H. Oliver in 1920. Dr. Oliver used IV hydrogen peroxide to treat Indian troops who were suffering from an influenza and pneumonia epidemic. The death rate was reported to be over 80% at that time. Dr. Oliver's results showed his IV hydrogen peroxide-treated cohort of 24 soldiers had a mortality rate of 48% compared to the 80% death rate from those treated with the usual care at that time.[60] In the article published by Dr. Oliver, he stated that the low oxygen symptoms his patients suffered from were markedly benefited by the use of intravenous hydrogen peroxide. Furthermore, he reported that the 'toxemia' (spread of bacterial products in the blood stream) appears to be overcome in many cases. Poor oxygenation and sepsis are both conditions experienced by **COVID-19** subjects.

When H_2O_2 is produced extracellularly or added to a cell culture system, a gradient of H_2O_2 is quickly established across the plasma membrane.[61] Researchers reported that the gradient is the result of H_2O_2-scavanging enzymes including catalase and GSH-peroxidase that maintains a steady-state intracellular H_2O_2 concentration being 10x less than the extracellular concentration.[62] As Bocci states, "This result is important because the intravenous (IV) infusion of a low and calculated concentration of H_2O_2 results in a marked dilution in the plasma pool with partial inactivation and in intracellular levels able to exert biological effects on blood and endothelial cells without aggravating the concomitant oxidative stress."[63] **COVID-19** is known to cause oxidative stress which may be the cause of multi organ failure and hypoxemia.[64][65][66] H_2O_2 is known to activate glycolysis, ATP and 2,3-DPG in red blood cells which can lead to improved oxygen delivery to ischemic tissues.[67][68] H_2O_2 has also been shown to increase the production of NO which can aid in vasodilation and tissue oxygenation.[69][70]

Researchers studying the effects of intravenous H_2O_2 therapy reported that it barely increases the plasma level of peroxidation end-products (lipid oxygenation products). This stimulates the production of antioxidants which act as reducing agents. The scientists report similar effects with ozone therapy. This results in an up-regulation of antioxidant enzymes (SOD, GSH-peroxidase, G-6PD) in erythrocytes which has been demonstrated *in-vivo*.[71] Coronaviruses have been shown to be sensitive to oxidizing disinfectants such as a 0.5% hydrogen peroxide solution used as a surface disinfectant.[72] It is well accepted that the response of the immune system is the production of pro-oxidants which are known to disinfect pathogens.[73]

4.8 IV Vitamin C (Ascorbate)

Intravenous use of vitamin C has been used in hospitals and outpatient settings for **COVID-19** patients after a report from China showed improvement in those treated with it.[74] IV ascorbic acid was introduced to moderately to severely sick **COVID-19** patients in Chinese hospitals. The researchers reported that intravenous ascorbic acid provided safe and effective adjunctive care of hospitalized **COVID-19** patients. There was no mortality, no reported side effects and shorter hospital stays universally. The Shanghai expert group recommends intravenous ascorbic acid use in extremely critical settings within **COVID-19** patients. In the US, multiple hospital centers utilized IV vitamin C to treat **COVID-19** patients.

We have been successfully utilizing IV vitamin C therapies for over two decades in order to aid the immune system in its ability to fight pathogens. For this study, we administered 2.5 gm of sodium ascorbate mixed with 5 cc of sterile water as an intravenous push over 1-2 minutes. There were no adverse effects from this regimen.

4.9 Intramuscular Ozone

Ozone is a colorless gas with a pungent odor. It is a natural molecule made up of three atoms of oxygen. Ozone is produced by an ozone generator where oxygen (O2) gas is exposed to an electrical discharge combining O2 molecules into a mixture of up to 5% O3 and 95% O2. Ozone therapy has been used for over 100 years and is widely used in

Europe and Cuba and in outpatient offices in the United States. Ozone has been used to treat infections and wounds as well as other illnesses over this time period. Ozone therapy can be administered by many different methods including intravenously and intramuscularly. Intramuscular ozone was given in these cases to reduce transmission risk. Since we were only treating **COVID-19** patients outside the office in the parking lot, intramuscular injections of ozone were deemed the easiest and safest modality.

IM ozone was provided to 37 patients (35%). Of these, a single ozone injection was given to 31 (82%). Seven (18%) required more than one IM injection. Five received two ozone shots, one patient had four and another had six. The patients who required four and six injections had been ill for a longer time period (over 10 days) before instituting therapy. Both recovered uneventfully. In viral infections, ozone has been shown to improve both the innate and adaptive immune systems while also reducing cytokine storm. Ozone improves neutrophil counts in children with compromised phagocyte cell-mediated immunity.[75] Antibodies have been shown to kill pathogens by producing ozone gas.[76] Ozone has been shown to have direct viricidal effects by disrupting the lipid envelope of a virus at sites of double bonds. When the lipid envelope is fragmented, its DNA or RNA cannot survive. **SARS-CoV-2** is an enveloped virus which would make it an excellent candidate for treatment with ozone.[77] Furthermore, **SARS-CoV-2**, as well as other coronaviruses, have abundant cysteine–a thiol containing amino acid– in their spike proteins. Rowen has hypothesized that ozone is the ideal therapy for viruses.[78] In order to successfully penetrate cell membranes, many viruses require membrane glycoproteins to be in the R-S-H reduced form as opposed to the oxidized—R-S-S-R– form. If virus thiol groups are oxidized they lose infectivity.[79] Rowen states, "Creating a more "oxidized" environment may allow ozone therapy…to assist the body in inactivating thiols in viruses in blood and tissues." **SARS-CoV-2** cell entry spike proteins are particularly rich in both cysteine and tryptophan the two most vulnerable amino acids to alteration by ozone.[80][81] The thiol group of cysteine is easily oxidized reversibly to disulfide which is widely accepted to neutralize the function of its protein/enzyme. Effectively, it is an "on-off" switch. Potent oxidants, such as hydrogen peroxide or ozone, can irreversibly oxidize the thiol. Regardless, viruses have no means to self-repair even when in the disulfide oxidation state. Regarding tryptophan, its electron rich indole group is very vulnerable to irreversible oxidation, even by hydrogen peroxide.[82] Ozone, like ascorbate, has been shown to increase the production of hydrogen peroxide.[83][84] This viral redox vulnerability theory was verified with the use of ozone rapidly remitting 100% of 5 cases of Ebola in 2014. The Ebola virus similarly has a large quantity of cysteine in its membrane glycoproteins.57 **COVID-19** is associated with microthrombotic events and, often, a cytokine storm of inflammation. Ozone could be particularly useful as it improves the prostacyclin:thromboxane ratio and enhances nitric oxide production.[85] Ozone has been shown to reduce production of TNF-α[86] as effectively as steroids do and increases the production of the anti-inflammatory enzyme heme oxygenase-1.[87] Ozone treatment also induces *Nrf 2* phosphorylation, which has been reported to reduce oxidative stress and proinflammatory cytokines in multiple sclerosis patients, and, in low doses.[88] *Nrf 2* is a regulator of genes related to antioxidant responses.[89] The limitations of this study include that most patients were taking nutritional supplements before they became ill. Therefore, they may have had fewer nutritional deficiencies compared to the average American. Furthermore, the majority of the subjects in this study, which mirrored the practice, were women. As compared to women, more men die of **COVID-19**.[90] Hypertension, diabetes, and obesity are known co-morbidities with **COVID-19**.[91] Our patient population had lower rates of these illnesses when compared to US averages. Since this was not a randomized, double-blind, placebo-controlled study, the therapies provided here cannot be proven to cure the symptoms of **COVID-19**. The observations of the positive outcomes are supported by this consecutive case

series even without a control group. During the **COVID-19** pandemic, we felt that it was not ethical to use a control group and withhold treatment from ill **COVID-19** patients.

Case control series have been shown to play an important role in evidence generation and in clinical practice.[92] The author of the fore worded report, Cynthia Jackevicius states, "Who better than clinicians who are the first to see how new therapies are being used and how patients respond to the new therapies—to share their valuable insights and experience in the medical literature through the use of case reports? A fundamental tenet of evidence-based clinical practice is to use the best available clinical evidence, and at times, a case report or case series is the best available evidence to guide decision-making."

Additionally, the results of this study offer a new consideration for the current medical study paradigm, which generally evaluates a single agent (or occasionally more) against a disease or pathogen. Considering the very favorable outcome of our consecutive case cohort (no deaths, only one hospitalization in patients treated prior to admission, and rapid recovery), this work supports an alternate paradigm for infection and medical challenges: providing support of the body's biochemical/nutritional needs and augmenting its innate physiological defense responses. Every substance used in our cohort is either an essential nutrient or an oxidant mediator actually manufactured by the body. Nothing foreign to the body was used, nor anything patentable. The disparity in the health outcomes under our treatment protocol and the outcomes in the rates of serious and critical illness and death under other protocols is stark and demands further investigation.

5. Conclusion

In summary, we treated 107 COVID-19 patients, solely with biological therapies, who all recovered. Only three were hospitalized. Of the three hospitalizations, two were hospitalized before beginning our treatment and sought our care post hospitalization. One was hospitalized while solely taking the oral regimen of Vitamins A, C, D, and iodine, and not the oxidative therapies. All recovered uneventfully. There were no deaths.

In the state of Michigan, as of 6/21/20, the case fatality rate was 9.0% (6,067 deaths and 67,097 positive cases of SARS-CoV-2). [92] Therefore, out of our 107 COVID-19 patients, 10 deaths could be predicted. At the very least, with 25 patients testing positive for the virus, we should have expected two deaths, but in reality, we should have seen significantly more morbidity considering we only had 33 tests performed on the 107 patients (all symptomatic), a median age of 56, and comorbid conditions. Of the 107 patients total, we should have experienced at least eight hospitalizations considering the median age, according to a published analysis. [93]

As of this publication, no cure, treatment, or preventive for SARS-CoV-2 has yet been proven effective in a randomized study, except for dexamethasone (a potent steroid) use in severely ill, hospitalized patients. In this study a novel treatment program, which is hypothesized to aid and support the immune system, was highly effective in the re-covery of 100% of 107 patients. This case review points out that specific and relatively inexpensive nutritional support along with oxidative intravenous as well as intramuscular, and nebulized oxidative solutions may be helpful for COVID-19 patients. Future, randomized studies are needed to elucidate the effectiveness of this or similar regimens.

6. Acknowledgments

The authors would like to acknowledgment Mark Rosner M.D. for his encouragement and help with the design of the study.

References

[1] MSN. **MSN covid tracker** . *MSN.com*, 2020. MSN coronavirus .

[2] Wertheim JO, Chu DK, Peiris JS, Kosakovsky Pond SL, and Poon LL. **A case for the ancient origin of coronaviruses** . *J Virol.*, 87(12):7039-7045, 2013. DOI .

[3] King A, Lefkowitz E, Adams M, and Carstens E. **Virus Taxonomy. 9th ed** . *Elsevier*, pages 806–828., 2011. Elsevier .

[4] Wertheim JO, Chu DK, Peiris JS, Kosakovsky Pond SL, and Poon LL. **A case for the ancient origin of coronaviruses** . *J Virol.*, 87(12):7039-7045, 2013. DOI .

[5] Peiris JSM, Lai ST, LLM Poon, Y Guan, LYC Yam, W Lim, J Nicholls, WKS Yee, WW Yan, MT Cheung, VCC Cheng, KH Chan, DNC Tsang, RWH Yung, TK Ng, and KY Yuen. **Coronavirus as a possible cause of severe acute respiratory syndrome** . *The Lancet*, 361(9366):1319–1325, 2003. The Lancet .

[6] Fehr A.R. and Perlman S. **Coronaviruses: An Overview of Their Replication and Pathogenesis. In: Maier H., Bickerton E., Britton P. (eds) Coronaviruses. Methods in Molecular Biology** . *Humana Press, New York, NY*, 1282, (2015). Springer .

[7] WHO EMRO. **MERS Outbreaks** . 2020. PubMed .

[8] Kristian G. Andersen, Andrew Rambaut, W. Ian Lipkin, Edward C. Holmes, and Robert F. Garr. **The proximal origin of SARS-CoV-2.** . *Nature Medicine*, (26):450–452, 2020. Nature Medicine .

[9] **Coronavirus (COVID-19) frequently asked questions.** . *Centers for Disease Control and Prevention*, June 2020. CDC .

[10] CDC. **Information for Healthcare Professionals about Coronavirus (COVID-19)** . *CDC*, 2020. CDC .

[11] Heidi Ledford. **Coronavirus breakthrough: dexamethasone is first drug shown to save lives** . *Nature*, JUne 2020. Nature .

[12] WHO. **Micronutrient Deficiencies** . *World Health Organization*, 2020. WHO .

[13] Eduardo Villamor and Wafaie W. Fawzi. **Vitamin A Supplementation: Implications for Morbidity and Mortality in Children** . *The Journal of Infectious Diseases*, 182:122–133, September 2000. Oxford .

[14] Osborne TB, Mendel LB, Ferry EL, and Wakeman AJ. **THE RELATION OF GROWTH TO THE CHEMICAL CONSTITUENTS OF THE DIET** . *Journal of Biological Chemistry*, 15:311–326, 1913. ☐.

[15] Green H. N. and Mellanby E.. . **VITAMIN A AS AN ANTI-INFECTIVE AGENT** . *Br Med J* , 2:691, 1928. PubMed Central .

[16] Villamor E and Fawzi WW. **Effects of Vitamin a supplementation on immune responses and correlation with clinical outcomes** . *Clin Microbiol Rev*, 18(3):446-464, 2005. PubMed .

[17] Freudenberg N., Freudenberg M.A., and Guzman J and et al. . **Identification of endotoxin-positive cells in the rat lung during shock** . *Vichows Archiv A Pathol Anat* , 404:197–211, 1984. DOI .

[18] Wong YC and Buck RC. **An electron microscopic study of metaplasia of the rat tracheal epithelium in Vitamin A deficiency** . *Lab Invest*, 24(1):55-66, 1971. PubMed .

[19] Wannee Rojanapo, Adrian J. Lamb, and James A. Olson. **The Prevalence, Metabolism and Migration of Goblet Cells in Rat Intestine following the Induction of Rapid, Synchronous Vitamin A Deficiency** . *The Journal of Nutrition*, 110(1):178–188, January 1980. DOI .

[20] Rosemary A. Warden, Marisa J. Strazzari, Peter R. Dunkley, and Edward V. O'Loughlin. **Vitamin A-Deficient Rats have Only Mild Changes in Jejunal Structure and Function** . *The Journal of Nutrition*, 126(7):1817–1826, July 1996. PubMed .

[21] Dillehay D, Walia A, and Lamon. **Effects of Retinoids on Macrophage Function and IL-1 Activity** . *J Leukoc Biol*, (44):353–360, 1988. DOI .

[22] Mehta P., McAuley D., Brown M., Sanchez E., Tattersall, R, and Manson J. **COVID-19: consider cytokine storm syndromes and immunosuppression** . *The Lancet*, 395(10229):1033–1034, 2020. PubMed .

[23] IBID Villamor E and Fawzi WW. **Effects of Vitamin a supplementation on immune responses and correlation with clinical outcomes** . *Clin Microbiol Rev*, 18(3):446-464, 2005. PubMed .

[24] Mehta P., McAuley D., Brown M., Sanchez E., Tattersall, R, and Manson J. **COVID-19: consider cytokine storm syndromes and immunosuppression** . *The Lancet*, 395(10229):1033–1034, 2020. PubMed .

[25] Wang D, Hu B, Hu C, and et al. **Clinical Characteristics of 138 Hospitalized Patients With 2019 Novel Coronavirus–Infected Pneumonia in Wuhan, China.** . *JAMA*, 323(11):1061–1069, 2020. PubMed .

[26] Mazanec and et al. **Intracellular neutralization of influenza virus by immunoglobulin A anti-hemagglutinin monoclonal antibodies** . *J. Virol*, 69:1339– 1343, 1995. PubMed Central .

[27] Mazanec et al. **Intracellular neutralization of Sendai and influenza viruses by IgA monoclonal antibodies** . *Adv. Exp. Med. Biol*, 371:651–654, 1995. Springer .

[28] Lamm Michael and et al. **IgA and mucosal defense.** . *APMIS: Journal of Pathology, Microbiology and Immunology*, January 1995. DOI .

[29] et al. Sterlin, Delphine. **IgA dominates the early neutralizing antibody response to SARS-CoV-2.** . 2020. DOI .

[30] Gangopadhyay NN, Moldoveanu Z, and Stephensen CB. **Vitamin A deficiency has different effects on immunoglobulin A production and transport during influenza A infection in BALB/c mice.** . *J Nutr.*, 126(12):2960-2967, 1996. DOI .

[31] Lie C, Ying C, Wang EL, Brun T, and Geissler C. **Impact of large-dose Vitamin A supplementation on childhood diarrhoea (sic), respiratory disease and growth.** . *Eur J Clin Nutr*, 47(2):88-96, 1993. PubMed .

[32] Shanghai new coronavirus disease clinical treatment expert group. **Shanghai 2019 coronavirus disease comprehensive treatment expert consensus** . *Journal of Infectious Diseases (Network Pre publishing)*, 38, May 2020. LINK .

[33] Fowler AA, Truwit JD, Hite RD, and et al. **Effect of Vitamin C Infusion on Organ Failure and Biomarkers of Inflammation and Vascular Injury in Patients With Sepsis and Severe Acute Respiratory Failure : The CITRIS-ALI Randomized Clinical Trial** . *JAMA*, 322(13):1261–1270, 2019. DOI .

[34] Chen L, Liu HG, Liu W, and et al. **Zhonghua Jie He He Hu Xi Za Zhi** . *Journal of Tuberculosis and Respiratory Diseases*, 43(0), Feb 2020. EuropePMC .

[35] Mohanty J., Nagababu E., and Rifkind J. **Red blood cell oxidative stress impairs oxygen delivery and induces red blood cell aging** . *Frontiers in Physiology*, 5, 2014. PubMed .

[36] Erol A. **High-dose intravenous Vitamin C treatment for COVID-19** . DOI .

[37] Lu P, Ma D, Yan C, Gong X, Du M, and Shi Y. **Structure and mechanism of a eukaryotic transmembrane ascorbate-dependent oxidoreductase** . *Proc Natl Acad Sci U S A*, 2014. DOI .

[38] Chen Q, Espey MG, Krishna MC, and et al. **Pharmacologic ascorbic acid concentrations selectively kill cancer cells: action as a pro-drug to deliver hydrogen peroxide to tissues** . *Proc Natl Acad Sci U S A*, 102(38):13604-13609, 2005. DOI .

[39] Alipio Mark. **Vitamin D Supplementation Could Possibly Improve Clinical Outcomes of Patients Infected with Coronavirus-2019 (COVID-19)** . April 2020. Abstract .

[40] J.I. Kast, A.J. McFarlane, A. Głobińska, M. Sokolowska, P. Wawrzyniak, M. Sanak, J. Schwarze, C.A. Akdis, and K. Wanke. **Respiratory syncytial virus infection influences tight junction integrity.** . *Clin Exp Immunol*, 190:351–359, 2017. DOI .

[41] Schwalfenberg GK. **A review of the critical role of Vitamin D in the functioning of the immune system and the clinical implications of Vitamin D deficiency** . *Mol Nutr Food Res*, 55(1):96-108, 2011. DOI .

[42] Sharifi A, Vahedi H, Nedjat S, Rafiei H, and Hosseinzadeh-Attar MJ. **Effect of single-dose injection of Vitamin D on immune cytokines in ulcerative colitis patients: a randomized placebo-controlled trial.** . *APMIS*, 127(10):681-687, 2019. DOI .

[43] Daneshkhah A, Agrawal V, Eshein A, Subramanian H, Roy H, and Backman V. **The Possible Role of Vitamin D in Suppressing Cytokine Storm and Associated Mortality in COVID-19Patients** . *preprint*, 2020. DOI .

[44] Hansdottir S, Monick MM, Hinde SL, Lovan N, Look DC, and Hunninghake GW. **Respiratory epithelial cells convert inactive Vitamin D to its active form: potential effects on host defense** . *J Immunol*, 181(10):7090-7099, 2008. DOI .

[45] Gombart AF. **its role in protection against infection** . *Future Microbiol.*, 4(9):1151-1165, 2009. DOI .

[46] CDC. **Second National Report On Biochemical Indicators Of Diet And Nutrition In The U.S. Population** . 2020. CDC .

[47] Caldwell K., Makhmudov A., Ely E., Jones R., and R. Wang. **Iodine Status of the U.S. Population National Health and Nutrition Examination Survey, 2005–2006 and 2007–2008** . *Thyroid*, 21(4):419–427, 2011. DOI .

[48] Kathleen L. Caldwell, Yi Pan, Mary E. Mortensen, Amir Makhmudov, Lori Merrill, and John Moye. . *Thyroid*, pages 927–937, Aug 2013. DOI .

[49] Weetman AP, McGregor AM, Campbell H, Lazarus JH, Ibbertson HK, and Hall R. **Iodide enhances IgG synthesis by human peripheral blood lymphocytes in vitro** . *Acta*

Endocrinol (Copenh), 103(2):210-215, 1983. DOI .

[50] Zel'tser ME. **Vliianie khronicheskogo de-fitsita ĭoda v ratsione na razvitie infekt-sionnogo protsessa [Effect of a chronic iodine deficit in the ration on the development of the infectious process]** . *Zh Mikrobiol Epidemiol Immunobiol.*, 0(9):116-119, 1975. PubMed .

[51] Venturi S and Venturi M. **Iodine, thymus, and immunity** . *Nutrition*, 25(9):977-979, 2009. DOI .

[52] Pelletier J., Tessema B., Westover J., Frank S., Brown S., and Capriotti J. **In Vitro Efficacy of Povidone-Iodine Nasal And Oral Antiseptic Preparations Against Severe Acute Respiratory Syndrome-Coronavirus 2 (SARS-CoV-2).** . *PrePrint*, 2020. PrePrint .

[53] Eggers M, Koburger-Janssen T, Eickmann M, and Zorn J. **In Vitro Bactericidal and Virucidal Efficacy of Povidone-Iodine Gargle/Mouthwash Against Respiratory and Oral Tract Pathogens** . *Infect Dis Ther*, 7(2):249-259, 2018. DOI .

[54] Abraham G., Flechas J, and Hakala J. **Orthoiodosupplementation: Iodine Sufficiency Of The Whole Human Body** . *Optimox.com*, 2020. OPTIMOX .

[55] Chance B, Sies H, and Boveris A. **Hydroperoxide metabolism in mammalian organs** . *Physiol Rev.*, 59(3):527-605, 1979. DOI .

[56] Halliwell Barry and Clement Marie Veronique and Long Lee Hua. **Hydrogen peroxide in the human body** . *FEBS Letters*, page 486, 2000. DOI .

[57] Rysz J, Stolarek RA, Luczynski R, and et al. **Increased hydrogen peroxide concentration in the exhaled breath condensate of stable COPD patients after nebulized N-acetylcysteine** . *Pulm Pharmacol Ther.*, 20(3):281-289, 2007. DOI .

[58] Zonta W, Mauroy A, Farnir F, and Thiry E. **Virucidal Efficacy of a Hydrogen Peroxide Nebulization Against Murine Norovirus and Feline Calicivirus, Two Surrogates of Human Norovirus** . *Food Environ Virol.*, 8(4):275-282, 2016. DOI .

[59] M Reth. **Hydrogen peroxide as second messenger in lymphocyte activation** . *Nat Immunol 3*, page 1129–1134, 2002. PubMed .

[60] Oliver T. and Murphy D. **INFLUENZAL PNEUMONIA : THE INTRAVENOUS INJECTION OF HYDROGEN PEROXIDE** . *The Lancet*, 195(5034):432–433, 1920. PDF .

[61] Antunes F. and Cadenas E. **Estimation of H2O2 gradients across biomembranes** . *FEBS Letters*, 475(2):121–126, 2000. PubMed .

[62] James R. Stone and Tucker Collins . **The Role of Hydrogen Peroxide in Endothelial Proliferative Responses** . *Endothelium*, 9(4):231–238, 2002 . DOI .

[63] Bocci V., Aldinucci Carlo, and Bianchi L. **The use of hydrogen peroxide as a medical drug** . *Rivista Italiana di Ossigeno-Ozonoterapia*, 4:30–39, 2005. PDF .

[64] Clinicaltrials.gov. **Correlation Between Oxidative Stress Status And COVID-19 Severity** . *Clinicaltrials.gov*, 2020 . ClinicalTrials .

[65] Zhang C, Wu Z, Li J, Zhao H, and Wang G. **Cytokine release syndrome in severe COVID-19: interleukin-6 receptor antagonist tocilizumab may be the key to reduce mortality** . *Int J Antimicrob Agents*, 55(5):105954, 2020. DOI .

[66] Menéndez R Bermejo-Martin J, Almansa R, Mendez R, Kelvin D, and Torres A. **Lymphopenic community acquired pneumonia as signature of severe COVID-19 infection** . *Journal of Infection*, 80(5):e23–e24, 2020. PubMed .

[67] Bocci V. **Oxygen-Ozone Therapy** . *Dordrecht: Springer*, page 1440, 2002. Springer .

[68] Bocci V. . **Ozone - A New Medical Drug 2nd ed. Dordrecht:** . *Springer Netherlands*, pages 1–295, 2011. Springer .

[69] Valacchi G and Bocci V. **Studies on the biological effects of ozone: 11. Release of factors from human endothelial cells** . *Mediators Inflamm.*, 9(6):271-276, 2000. DOI .

[70] Thengchaisri N and Kuo L. **Hydrogen peroxide induces endothelium-dependent and -independent coronary arteriolar dilation: role of cyclooxygenase and potassium channels** . *American Journal of Physiology-Heart and Circulatory Physiology*, 285(6):H2255–H2263, 2003. DOI .

[71] IBID. Bocci V, Aldinucci Carlo, and Bianchi L. **The use of hydrogen peroxide as a medical drug** . *Rivista Italiana di Ossigeno-Ozonoterapia*, 4:30–39, 2005. PDF .

[72] Kampf G, Todt D, Pfaender S, and Steinmann E. **Persistence of coronaviruses on inanimate surfaces and their inactivation with biocidal agents** . *Journal of Hospital Infection*, 104(3):246–251, 2020. DOI .

[73] Aaron J. Smith, John Oertle, Dan Warren, and Dino Prato. **Ozone Therapy: A Critical Physiological and Diverse Clinical Evaluation with Regard to Immune Modulation, Anti-Infectious Properties, Anti-Cancer Potential, and Impact on Anti-Oxidant Enzymes** . *Open Journal of Molecular and Integrative Physiology*, 5(3):37–48, 2015. DOI .

[74] IBID. **Shanghai new coronavirus disease clinical treatment expert group. Shanghai 2019 coronavirus disease comprehensive treatment expert consensus.** . *Journal of Infectious Diseases*, 38, 3 2020. LINK .

[75] Díaz LJ, Sardiñas PG, Menéndez CS, and et al. **Immunomodulator effect of ozone therapy in children with deficiency in immunity mediated by phagocytes** . *Mediciego*, 18(1), 2012. Medigraphic .

[76] Wentworth P. Evidence for Antibody-Catalyzed. **Ozone Formation in Bacterial Killing and Inflammation** . *Science*, 298(5601):2195–2199, 2002. DOI .

[77] Walter LA and McGregor AJ. **Sex- and Gender-specific Observations and Implications for COVID-19.** . *West J Emerg Med.*, 21(3):507-509, Apr 2020. DOI .

[78] Rowen RJ. **Ozone and oxidation therapies as a solution to the emerging crisis in infectious disease management: a review of current knowledge and experience** . *Med Gas Res.*, 9(4):232-237, 2019. DOI .

[79] Mirazimi A, Mousavi-Jazi M, Sundqvist VA, and Svensson L. **Free thiol groups are essential for infectivity of human cytomegalovirus** . *J Gen Virol*, 80(Pt 11):2861-2865, 1999. DOI .

[80] Broer R, Boson B, Spaan W, Cosset FL, and Corver J. **Important role for the transmembrane domain of severe acute respiratory syndrome coronavirus spike protein during entry** . *J Virol.*, 80(3):1302-1310, 2006. PubMed .

[81] Virender K. Sharma and Nigel J.D. Graham . **Oxidation of Amino Acids, Peptides and Proteins by Ozone: A Review, Ozone** . *Science & Engineering*, 32(2):81–90, 2010 . DOI .

[82] KUNAPULI S, KHAN N, DIVAKAR N, and VAIDYANATHAN C. **OXIDATION OF INDOLES** . *Journal of the Indian Institute of Science*, 2020. LINK .

[83] IBID. Bocci V. **Oxygen-Ozone Therapy** . *Dordrecht: Springer*, 1440, 2002. Springer .

[84] IBID. Bocci V, Aldinucci Carlo, and Bianchi L. **The use of hydrogen peroxide as a medical drug** . *Rivista Italiana di Ossigeno-Ozonoterapia*, 4:30–39, 2005. PDF .

[85] Schulz S, Ninke S, Watzer B, and Nüsing RM. **Ozone induces synthesis of systemic prostacyclin by cyclooxygenase-2 dependent mechanism in vivo** . *Biochem Pharmacol*, 83(4):506-513, 2012. DOI .

[86] Zamora ZB, Borrego A, López OY, and et al. **Effects of ozone oxidative preconditioning on TNF-alpha release and antioxidant-prooxidant intracellular balance in mice during endotoxic shock** . *Mediators Inflamm,* 2005(1):16-22, 2005. DOI .

[87] Pecorelli A, Bocci V, Acquaviva A, and et al. **NRF2 activation is involved in ozonated human serum upregulation of HO-1 in endothelial cells** . *Toxicol Appl Pharmacol,* 267(1):30-40, 2013. DOI .

[88] Delgado-Roche L, Riera-Romo M, , Mesta F, Hernández-Matos Y, Barrios J, and et al. **Medical ozone promotes Nrf2 phosphorylation reducing oxidative stress and proinflammatory cytokines in multiple sclerosis patients** . *Eur J Pharm,* 811:148–154, 2017. PubMed .

[89] Ma Q. **Role of Nrf2 in Oxidative Stress and Toxicity** . *Annu Rev Pharmacol Toxicol,* 53:401–426 , 2013. DOI .

[90] Lancet Staff. **The gendered dimensions of COVID-19** . *The Lancet,* 395(10231):1168, 2020. DOI .

[91] Yang J, Zheng Y, Gou X, and et al. **Prevalence of comorbidities and its effects in patients infected with SARS-CoV-2: a systematic review and meta-analysis** . *Int J Infect Dis,* 94:91-95, 2020. DOI .

[92] Jackevicius Cynthia. **The Value of Case Reports** . *Can. J. Hosp. Pharm.,* 71(6):345–6, Nov-Dec 2018. PubMed Central .

[93] Verity R and et.al. **Estimates of the severity of coronavirus disease 2019: a model-based analysis** . *Lancet Journal of Infectious diseases,* 20(6):669–677 , 2020. The Lancet .

***Editor's Erratum Note, 7/9/2020, 8:20PM
Due to a typographical error, the amount of Vitamin A in the protocol was originally reported as 10,000 IU/day. The correct value should have been 100,000 IU/day.

Index

Vitamin D 9, 32, 45, 89-103,
109, 177, 123
Vitamin E 68

X

Y

Z

Books by David Brownstein, M.D.
More information: www.drbrownstein.com

The Statin Disaster
Statin drugs are the most profitable drugs in the history of Big Pharma. The best of the studies show statin drugs fail to significantly lower your risk of developing heart disease. This book will tell you the truth about statin drugs. Statins are associated with a host of adverse effects including:

- ALS
- Breast Cancer
- Congestive Heart Failure
- Memory Loss

- *Myopathy*
- *Neuropathy*
- *Sexual Dysfunction*
- *Skin Cancer*

Vitamin B12 for Health
Vitamin B12 deficiency is occurring in epidemic numbers. This book show you the many benefits of using natural, bioidentical forms of vitamin B12 and how B12 supplements can help you achieve your optimal health. B12 therapy can treat many common ailments including:

- Anemia
- Autoimmune Illness
- Blood Clots
- Brain Fog
- Cognitive Decline

- Depression
- Fatigue
- Fibromyalgia
- Heart Disease
- Muscle Disease

- Neurologic Problems
- Osteoporosis
- AND MUCH MORE!

IODINE: WHY YOU NEED IT, WHY YOU CAN'T LIVE WITHOUT IT, 5th EDITION
Iodine is the most misunderstood nutrient. Dr. Brownstein shows you the benefit of supplementing with iodine. Iodine deficiency is rampant. It is a world-wide problem and is at near epidemic levels in the United States. Most people wrongly assume that you get enough iodine from iodized salt. Dr. Brownstein convincingly shows you why it is vitally important to get your iodine levels measured. He shows you how iodine deficiency is related to:

- Breast cancer
- Hypothyroidism and Graves' disease
- Autoimmune illnesses
- Chronic Fatigue and Fibromyalgia
- Cancer of the prostate, ovaries, and much more!

OVERCOMING ARTHRITIS

Dr. Brownstein shows you how a holistic approach can help you overcome arthritis, fibromyalgia, chronic fatigue syndrome, and other conditions. This approach encompasses the use of:

- Allergy elimination
- Detoxification
- Diet
- Natural, bioidentical hormones
- Vitamins and minerals
- Water

DRUGS THAT DON'T WORK and
NATURAL THERAPIES THAT DO, 2nd Edition

Dr. Brownstein's newest book will show you why the most commonly prescribed drugs may not be your best choice. Dr. Brownstein shows why drugs have so many adverse effects. The following conditions are covered in this book: high cholesterol levels, depression, GERD and reflux esophagitis, osteoporosis, inflammation, and hormone imbalances. He also gives examples of natural substances that can help the body heal.

See why the following drugs need to be avoided:

- Cholesterol-lowering drugs (statins such as Lipitor, Zocor, Mevacor, and Crestor and Zetia)
- Antidepressant drugs (SSRI's such as Prozac, Zoloft, Celexa, Paxil)
- Antacid drugs (H-2 blockers and PPI's such as Nexium, Prilosec, and Zantac)
- Osteoporosis drugs (Bisphosphonates such as Fosomax and Actonel, Zometa, and Boniva)
- Diabetes drugs (Metformin, Avandia, Glucotrol, etc.)
- Anti-inflammatory drugs (Celebrex, Vioxx, Motrin, Naprosyn, etc)
- Synthetic Hormones (Provera and Estrogen)

SALT YOUR WAY TO HEALTH , 2nd Edition

Dr. Brownstein dispels many of the myths of salt—salt is bad for you, salt causes hypertension. These are just a few of the myths Dr. Brownstein tackles in this book. He shows you how the right kind of salt--unrefined salt--can have a remarkable health benefit to the body. Refined salt is a toxic, devitalized substance for the body. Unrefined salt is a necessary ingredient for achieving your optimal health. See how adding unrefined salt to your diet can help you:

- Maintain a normal blood pressure
- Balance your hormones
- Optimize your immune system
- Lower your risk for heart disease

THE MIRACLE OF NATURAL HORMONES, 3rd EDITION

Optimal health cannot be achieved with an imbalanced hormonal system. Dr. Brownstein's research on bioidentical hormones provides the reader with a plethora of information on the benefits of balancing the hormonal system with bioidentical, natural hormones.

- Arthritis and autoimmune disorders
- Chronic fatigue syndrome and fibromyalgia
- Heart disease
- Hypothyroidism
- Menopausal symptoms

OVERCOMING THYROID DISORDERS, 3rd Edition

This book provides new insight into why thyroid disorders are frequently undiagnosed and how best to treat them. Detoxification

- Diet
- Graves'
- Hashimoto's Disease
- Hypothyroidism

Ozone: The Miracle Therapy

Ozone is one of the most exciting and effective medical therapies. This book will show you why ozone therapy should be taught in all medical schools. The medical uses of ozone are many and include:

- Increases oxygen delivery to tissues
- Kills bacteria, viruses, parasites, and fungi
- Stimulates cartilage to grow
- Enhances stem cell production
- And, much more!

THE GUIDE TO HEALTHY EATING, 2nd Edition

Which food do you buy? Where to shop? How do you prepare food? This book will answer all of these questions and much more. This book contains recipes and information on how best to feed your family. See how eating a healthier diet can help you:

- Avoid chronic illness
- Enhance your immune system

THE GUIDE TO A GLUTEN-FREE DIET, 2nd Edition

What would you say if 16% of the population (1/6) had a serious, life-threatening illness that was being diagnosed correctly only 3% of the time? Gluten-sensitivity is the most frequently missed diagnosis in the U.S. Why you should become gluten-free.

- Autoimmune disease and thyroid disorders

THE GUIDE TO A DAIRY-FREE DIET

This book will show you why dairy is not a healthy food. This book will dispel the myth that dairy from pasteurized milk is a healthy food choice. In fact, it is a devitalized food source which needs to be avoided.

- Osteoporosis
- Diabetes
- Allergies
- Asthma
- A Poor Immune System

THE SOY DECEPTION

This book will dispel the myth that soy is a healthy food. Soy ingestion can cause a myriad of severe health issues.

- Thyroid Disorders
- A Poor Immune System

The Skinny on Fats

The Skinny on Fat was written to educate you about the importance of consuming good sources of dietary fat. This book will teach you why we need fat and why we can't live without it.

- Prevent heart disease
- Promote weight loss
- Help prevent chronic illness

Call 1-888-647-5616 or
send a check or money order
BOOKS $20 each!

Sales Tax: For Michigan residents, please add $1.20 per book.

Shipping :	1-3 Books:	$5.00
	4-6 Books:	$4.00
	7-9 Books:	$3.00

Order 10 or more books: FREE SHIPPING!
VOLUME DISCOUNTS AVAILABLE. CALL
1-888-647-5616 FOR MORE INFORMATION
DVD's of Dr. Brownstein's Lectures Available! DVD's: $25.00 each
INFORMATION OR ORDER ON-LINE AT:
WWW.DRBROWNSTEIN.COM

You can send a check to: Medical Alternatives Press
4054 Oak Bank Ct.
Orchard Lake, MI 48323